Working with Vulnerable Groups

Working with Vulnerable Groups
A clinical handbook for GPs

Edited by Paramjit Gill, Nat Wright and Iain Brew

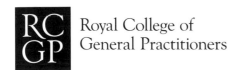

Royal College of
General Practitioners

The Royal College of General Practitioners was founded in 1952 with this object:

'To encourage, foster and maintain the highest possible standards in general practice and for that purpose to take or join with others in taking steps consistent with the charitable nature of that object which may assist towards the same.'

Among its responsibilities under its Royal Charter the College is entitled to:

'Diffuse information on all matters affecting general practice and issue such publications as may assist the object of the College.'

....

British Library Cataloguing-in-Publication Data
A catalogue record for this book is available from the British Library

© Royal College of General Practitioners, 2014
Published by the Royal College of General Practitioners, 2014
30 Euston Square, London NW1 2FB

Designed and typeset by Typographic Design Unit

Printed by Charlesworth Press

Indexed by Susan Leech

ISBN: 978-0-85084-350-7

Disclaimer

This publication is intended for the use of medical practitioners in the UK and not for patients. The authors, editors and publisher have taken care to ensure that the information contained in this book is correct to the best of their knowledge, at the time of publication. Whilst efforts have been made to ensure the accuracy of the information presented, particularly that related to the prescription of drugs, the authors, editors and publisher cannot accept liability for information that is subsequently shown to be wrong. Readers are advised to check that the information, especially that related to drug usage, complies with information contained in the *British National Formulary*, or equivalent, or manufacturers' datasheets, and that it complies with the latest legislation and standards of practice.

Contents

Foreword

In *A Fortunate Man*, his defining portrait of a GP, John Berger wrote: 'Vulnerability may have its own private causes, but it often reveals concisely what is wounding and damaging on a much larger scale.'[1] As contemporary political ideology drives ever increasing socioeconomic polarisation of society, this wounding and damaging proceeds apace. The extent of inequality has become profoundly disturbing. To take London as an example, the '90:10 ratio' for wealth in the UK's capital city, which was already high (at 199) in 2006/8, had risen even higher by 2010 (to 215). This means that the poorest person of the richest 10% of the population consumes 215 times as much as the richest person of the poorest 10%.[2] This was in 2010 and, with the imposition of austerity measures and sweeping cuts to welfare benefits, it is almost certainly worse by now. This is what economics Nobel laureate Joseph Stiglitz has described as 'trickle up' as opposed to the pipe dream of 'trickle down' that was supposed to follow from allowing the rich free reign to make more money.[3]

We have learned from the exhaustive work of Richard Wilkinson and Kate Pickett[4] of the Equality Trust that greater socioeconomic inequality is associated with a whole raft of health and social problems including lower social mobility, lower life expectancy, higher rates of teenage pregnancy, higher rates of obesity, higher infant mortality, more murders, a larger prison population, a higher proportion of the population living on less than 50% of median income, lower voting rates and lower reported trust in others. Inequality wounds and damages, and makes individuals and families vulnerable. As the situation worsens, GPs face ever greater challenges in caring for vulnerable groups and hence the importance of this book.

El-Kabir and Ramsden wrote concerning the primary health care of single homeless people: 'In many ways the consultation is the doctor's moment of truth where his authenticity, humanity, understanding, knowledge and intentions are put to the test.'[5] I have a friend, Harald Sundby, who is a wonderful GP in Norway and who describes the care of

---

1 Berger J, Mohr J. *A Fortunate Man*. Harmondsworth: Allen Lane, Penguin Press, 1967.

2 Lupton R, Vizard P, Fitzgerald A, *et al*. *Prosperity, Poverty and Inequality in London 2000/01–2010/11*. London: Centre for Analysis of Social Exclusion, LSE, 2013.

3 www.youtube.com/watch?v=wputRsxArSI [accessed October 2013].

4 Wilkinson R, Pickett K. *The Spirit Level: why equality is better for everyone*. London: Allen Lane, 2009.

5 El-Kabir D, Ramsden S. Primary healthcare of the single homeless. In: D Bhugra (ed.). *Homelessness and Mental Health*. Cambridge: Cambridge University Press, 1996.

patients with multiple vulnerabilities as 'extreme general practice' on a par with extreme sport and the arena within which he tests himself to his limits. He finds that it is in caring for these patients that he learns most: about his patients, about society and about himself. He identifies our complex marginalised and vulnerable patients as our true professors of general practice. Harald adds that extreme general practice, just like extreme sport, should never be done entirely alone. Emotional support is essential but it is also important not to believe entirely in the uniqueness of one's own commitment and achievement, and most of us need others around us to hold on to the necessary humility.

The care of vulnerable groups requires much more than technical skill. It calls for all the attributes of vocational professionalism, including a willingness to hear the true nature and extent of the patient's suffering. It requires too an acknowledgement of the patient's own values and aspirations, and the meaning ascribed to the illness within the context of a unique and often intensely damaging life story. Working this close to the vulnerability of others can very readily invoke our own and this is a large part of the challenge of 'extreme general practice'. As Howard Brody writes in *Stories of Sickness*:

> just as to be sick is to sense an unpleasant disruption of the self–body unity, to perceive sickness or disability in others is to be reminded of one's own vulnerability and mortality in an equally unpleasant and threatening way. Thus much reaction to sickness that superficially appears to be solely outward-directed (that is, towards meeting the needs of the sick person) is in reality also inner-directed as an attempt to remove, resolve, or transcend this inner threat to integrity.[6]

This perhaps explains why many doctors and other health professionals find working with vulnerable groups to be particularly difficult and even try to avoid it. My hope is that this book will make it easier for all doctors to engage in the care of those patients who need our care most and to realise the intense rewards both personal and professional that can result.

The care of those rendered vulnerable by the ways in which power is exercised and society is organised also carries a responsibility for advocacy and for interceding with the powerful on behalf of the relatively powerless. When the independence of doctors is eroded, as happens within totalitarian regimes and is happening now within contemporary technocratic and market-driven societies, important elements of civil

---

6 Brody H. *Stories of Sickness*. New Haven: Yale University Press, 1987.

power and societal justice are suppressed to the detriment of all.

In 2012, I had the privilege to attend a meeting organised by Pride in Practice. Asked to summarise how to provide excellence in lesbian, gay and bisexual health care, Paul Martin, the Chief Executive, replied: 'Be kind; don't judge; don't assume.' These are important words to bring to our lives and to our work with all of our patients, but perhaps particularly to our work with vulnerable groups.

Iona Heath CBE FRCGP
Past President of the Royal College of General Practitioners

Preface

'Vulnerable' indicates an inability to cope with a hostile environment. Life can be hostile for all of us, but members of 'vulnerable groups' may not have been lucky enough to develop the coping mechanisms needed for everyday living.

Some may have been born with physical or mental health problems, some may have suffered abuse in their formative years, and some have developed difficulties such as dementia later in life and have lost their ability to cope. Some are marginalised by society because they chose different lifestyles or cultures.

Any one of these groups may find mainstream everyday life difficult to deal with and may turn to drugs, alcohol or crime to get by. Such behaviour is likely to result in contact with the Criminal Justice System, leading in turn to further marginalisation, thus compounding the difficulties they face.

This book is for those who feel that working in primary care despite all its rigours and stresses is a privilege. If like the chapter authors you wish to better help those presenting in primary care as vulnerable but feel as if you sometimes lack the necessary knowledge and skills required, then this book is for you. It aims to guide the reader towards a better understanding of a variety of vulnerable groups so that the care we offer may be more tailored to their needs. This will allow the reader to offer help that is more useful and effective than that offered by the well-motivated generic practitioner.

Paramjit Gill, Nat Wright and Iain Brew

Contributors

Editors

Dr Paramjit Gill DM FRCGP is a GP in Birmingham and RCGP Clinical Champion for Social Inclusion. He is also reader in Primary Care Research at the University of Birmingham. His research interests include addressing inequalities in health and health care, particularly amongst migrant populations, and evidence-based health care and its application to healthcare delivery. He is a founding member of the RCGP Health Inequalities Standing Group and editor of the 'Promoting Equality and Valuing Diversity' e-GP learning module. He led on the *Improving Access to Health Care for Gypsies and Travellers, Homeless People and Sex Workers* commissioning guide.

Dr Nat Wright PhD FRCGP is the Clinical Director for Vulnerable Groups at NHS Leeds. He has worked with drug users for almost 20 years in both community primary care and secure-environment settings. Between 2003 and 2010 he held various positions as a government GP adviser with a remit to support GPs working in both mainstream primary care and secure environments. He is a regular contributor to the development of national and international guidelines pertaining to the care of drug users. He is currently a member of the RCGP Substance Misuse Unit Executive Committee and also the RCGP Secure Environments Group. He is also the clinical lead for the RCGP Certificate in Substance Misuse Part 2 course. From 2003–8 he was the Chair of the RCGP Health Inequalities Standing Group. He has published extensively on issues relating to the care of drug users.

Dr Iain Brew FRCGP has worked in challenging environments throughout his career. After five years as a GP in Shetland, he worked in oncology before returning to primary care in Lincoln. He was redeployed to HMP Lincoln, where he discovered his niche. Twelve years later, Iain is an established GP working with the most vulnerable members of society. He has a special interest in the treatment of hepatitis C in primary care and is passionate about improving patient safety. Iain's long-suffering wife Lisa is a fellow Birkonian and is his constant source of support.

Contributing authors

Dr A. Gordon Baird MRCOG FRCGP was a rural GP from 1980 until 2011. A founder member and later Chair of the RCGP Rural Practice Standing Group, he has published on rural health, with a particular interest in the effect rurality has on health inequalities. Papers include inequities in care provision for rural cancer patients, the misconceptions surrounding deprivation in rural areas and the challenges faced by poor socioeconomic groups in rural areas. He also described the first identified case of Lyme disease in Scotland, proved the endemic nature of the disease and researched the risks involved in the provision of low-risk maternity care. He is an enthusiastic yachtsman and has won the Scottish Islands Peaks Race on four occasions.

Dr Dick Churchill DM FRCGP is a part-time GP and Clinical Associate Professor and Director of Clinical Skills at the University of Nottingham Medical School. He is a past Chair of the RCGP Adolescent Health Group with whom he worked for a number of years. Dick has undertaken research into adolescent health and mental health in primary care, contributed to the development of training materials for GPs and practices, and has represented the RCGP on children's and young people's health issues nationally. He was a founder trustee of the Association for Young People's Health and also a co-editor of the e-Learning for Healthcare Adolescent Health Programme.

Prof. Jan De Maeseneer MD PhD FRCGP (Hon.) is Head of the Department of Family Medicine and Primary Health Care at Ghent University, and works part time as a GP. His research focuses on health inequities, education of health professionals, multimorbidity and global health. In 2004, he received the Wonca Five-Star Doctor Award for Excellence in Health Care. He contributed to the Knowledge Network on 'Health Systems' of the WHO Commission on Social Determinants of Health. He is the Chairman of the European Forum for Primary Care (www.euprimarycare.org) and the Secretary-General of the Network: Towards Unity for Health (www.the-networktufh.org). He is the Director of the International Center for Family Medicine and Primary Health Care at Ghent University, a WHO collaborating center on primary health care.

Dr Gilles de Wildt MSc MD MRCGP is a GP partner at Jiggins Lane Medical Centre and a Lecturer in International Health at the University of Birmingham. Previously, he worked in the Netherlands and Southern Africa in hospital care and public health. He has been a member of the RCGP Health Inequalities Standing Group since 1998 and co-edited, with Paramjit Gill, a book on housing, health and primary care. Gilles is a Trustee of Medact, an educational and health policy charity that is 'Challenging barriers to health'. He has published on health, trade and other economic policies, and has represented non-governmental organisations on these issues at meetings of UN organisations and other international events.

Dr Rayah Feldman DPhil has worked on refugee health issues for ten years after a career teaching social sciences and development studies. She currently works with the charity Maternity Action, where she wrote *Guidance for Commissioning Health Services for Vulnerable Migrant Women* and *When Maternity Doesn't Matter: dispersing pregnant women seeking asylum*. In 2006 she published a review of primary care services for refugees and asylum seekers in *Public Health*. She also campaigns on migrants' rights locally and is a co-founder of Hackney Migrant Centre.

Dr Angela Jones trained in medical sciences at Girton College, Cambridge, and completed her clinical training at Oxford in 1983. After a spell in paediatrics and vocational training as a GP, she was a full-time principal in South Wales before returning to Oxford. Locuming at the pioneering homeless medical centre in Luther Street opened up a whole new world of primary care, which she developed into a specialist interest. A wish to support co-workers in the field led to teaching, speaking and government advisory roles. She was co-founder of a European network for homeless health workers and a past Chair of the RCGP Health Inequalities Standing Group.

Prof. Una Macleod PhD FRCGP FHEA is Professor of Primary Care Medicine at the Hull York Medical School and works as a GP in Hull. She previously worked in Glasgow as a GP and academic, and has research interests in cancer in primary care and health inequalities. She chairs the RCGP's Health Inequalities Standing Group.

Dr Graham Martin MD FRCGP is past Chair of the RCGP Intellectual Disabilities Working Group. He was a full-time GP principal at Red Roofs Surgery, Nuneaton, Warwickshire from 1974 to 1998, and for some of that time was a GP trainer and course organiser. Graham wrote two RCGP e-learning modules and was previously guardian for the learning disabilities section of the RCGP curriculum. He is a member of the British Institute of Learning Disabilities and of Mencap, and has a son who has a profound learning disability. He is currently a member of the RCGP Intellectual Disabilities Professional Network and is Intellectual Disabilities Lead on the RCGP Health Inequalities Standing Group.

Dr Nwakuru Nwaogwugwu BSc MRCGP DFSRH is a sessional GP in Peckham, South London. She has an interest in vulnerable groups and also aids in the clinical care of migrants and refugees in a local outreach clinic. She enjoys voluntary work and has worked with the Medical Foundation and Project London in the UK and Evangelistic Medical Missions Abroad (EMMA) during a medical outreach to Kenya. In her current voluntary role she is trainee rep for the Medical Association of Nigerian Doctors Across GB (MANSAG) and is responsible for their mentoring and clinical attachment programme. She looks forward to her next, hopefully international, opportunity.

Dr Joseph O'Neill MRCGP is a retired GP. He was a consultant in palliative medicine and lectured in health inequalities at the University of Liverpool's Medical School.

Prof. Louise Robinson MD FRCGP is an academic GP in Newcastle upon Tyne and the RCGP Clinical Champion for Dementia. As Professor of Primary Care and Ageing at Newcastle University, she leads a research programme focused on improving quality of life and quality of care for older people, especially those with dementia. She is the national primary care representative on the Prime Minister's Dementia Challenge Health and Social Care Group and was part of the expert team who developed the Department of Health GP Commissioning Toolkits for dementia care. She has co-authored the BMJ Learning e-learning module on dementia in primary care.

Dr Paul Shire MRCGP started his GP career in Lewisham, South London, working in an area with high levels of social deprivation, sexually transmitted infections and a large migrant community. He is now working in Australia and has developed an interest in improving nutrition and diabetes care in disadvantaged groups.

Dr Surinder Singh BM MSc FRCGP is a Senior Lecturer at University College London (UCL) and a GP with a longstanding interest in HIV and AIDS. He is a senior partner in a thriving practice in Deptford, London, which is an area known for its typical inner-city challenges. He is also the course director for the Integrated BSc in Primary Health Care within the Research Department of Primary Care and Population Health at UCL. He has published on primary care and HIV/AIDS and on the multidisciplinary care of patients with HIV/AIDS, and is co-editor of *HIV in Primary Care* (MEDFASH publications). He is a former Chairman of the RCGP's Working Group on HIV and Sexual Health (1995–8) and was a member of the Independent Working Group on Sexual Health and HIV (2003–7).

Dr Rafik Taibjee MRCGP is a GP principal and GP trainer in South London, and a Programme Director of King's GP Training Scheme. He is Co-Chair of the UK Gay and Lesbian Association of Doctors and Dentists (GLADD) and the Chair of the BMA Equality and Diversity Committee. He currently is an adviser to the Terrence Higgins Trust, and sits on the NHS England Clinical Reference Group for Gender Identity Services. His greatest passion is providing education and training on lesbian, gay, bisexual and trans* (LGBT) health inequalities, having published research on healthy lifestyles and sexual risk-taking behaviour.

Dr Gervase Vernon MSc MRCP FRCGP DCH DRCOG is a retired GP in Essex. He worked as a Medical Examiner at Freedom from Torture from 2002 to 2011. He has published regularly in the BJGP, mainly on refugee issues.

Prof. Sara Willems MA PhD is an Associate Professor of Equity in Health Care at the Department of Family Medicine and General Practice at Ghent University in Belgium where she leads the Equity in Health Care Research Group. The work of this interdisciplinary group focuses on equity in (primary) health care, from the macro-level (comparing equity in European healthcare systems) to the micro-level (impact of practice organisation on equity of care, social gradient in the interaction between physician and patient). Sara is also lecturer on health equity, equity in health care and qualitative research in the Faculty of Medicine and Health Sciences at Ghent University. She is president of the board of Community Health Centre Watersportbaan, located in a deprived area in Ghent.

1 General practice, health inequalities and social exclusion

Una Macleod and Paramjit Gill

Key learning points

- Recognise the impact of health inequalities on health and health care.

- Understand the term 'social exclusion'.

- Describe the role of general practice in addressing health inequalities.

- Discuss the ethical issues raised in delivering care to disadvantaged groups.

Since the beginning of the NHS, inequalities in health have existed. Though a number of initiatives to tackle these have been described, health inequalities still remain a challenge. General practice is a core element of the new NHS and its role in tackling these inequalities is likely to increase in the coming years. This chapter provides an overview of the range of health inequalities and the role of general practice in addressing these.

First, we need to understand what the term 'social exclusion' means. For years policymakers have been speaking about health inequalities and disadvantage, and during the past decade social exclusion has become the preferred term. It refers to the inability of an individual, group or community to participate effectively in economic, social, political and cultural life: alienation and distance from the mainstream society.[1] It is a very broad definition and refers to people who are suffering multiple and enduring disadvantage; they do not have the opportunities that the majority of us take for granted. It can therefore include, for example, the homeless, asylum seekers and refugees. Can you think of any more groups?

Box 1.1 (overleaf) lists some further examples but note that this is not an exhaustive list and the groups can overlap with individuals having multiple complex health and social needs. The challenges of caring for some of these groups within general practice are covered in this book but first we provide the background to these.

> ### Box 1.1 **Examples of some socially excluded groups**
>
> - Asylum seekers and refugees.
> - Homeless.
> - People with learning disabilities.
> - People with physical disabilities.
> - Travellers.
> - Sex workers.
> - People living in remote rural areas.
> - Older people.
> - Young adults.
> - Offenders and ex-offenders.
> - Those in severe and persistent poverty.
> - Long-term unemployed.

The essence of general practice

The fundamental element of general practice is the relationship between patient and doctor. This remains true despite the considerable changes to society and to practice that have occurred over previous decades. In the past, this relationship was characterised by the term 'family doctor': GPs occupied a place in communities and in families, and continuity of care for patients by the same family doctor was the norm. Although this model has largely disappeared, the relationship between patient and GP is still key to modern health care. Continuity of care continues to be important, although this may sometimes be informational rather than personal. In some instances the relationship may be one that spans many years, while in others it may be for the duration of an episode of illness. For some patients it is a relationship with one doctor, while for others it is an ongoing engagement with a practice.

Traditionally, the doctor–patient relationship was based on face-to-face engagements lasting around 5–10 minutes (lengthening in more recent decades). More recently, other types of consultation have become more common, such as those via telephone and electronic communication. But regardless of method, at the heart of the process remains the encounter between patient and doctor. However, it is not only the type of consultation that has changed in recent years, but also the encounter itself, which has become increasingly complex. Whereas previously the GP–patient consultation was largely a diagnostic or supportive encounter, the general practice consultation may now also include health improvement and risk assessment, anticipatory care, long-term disease management, and advanced care planning. Similarly, the external pressures on GPs have also changed. Although many in the UK remain independent contractors, they are much more accountable to Primary Care Organisations and to professional bodies, a situation that adds its own weight to the doctor–patient encounter. For example, in many areas of the UK there are explicit pressures on drug and prescription budgets that need to be considered within the context of the individual consultation.

As well as caring for individual patients, GPs also take on a population perspective in managing conditions within the practice.[2] For example, procedures such as cardiovascular screening are initiated within practices to reduce the public health impact on a locality. Another example is working with other practices within a locality to ensure that services such as health visiting are provided.

Whatever the method of consultation, and regardless of internal or external influences, many GPs would describe good general practice as seeking to do the best for the individual patient in the consultation at any given point in time. This book challenges us to consider that all of our patients are not equal in terms of need, and that therefore we may have greater responsibilities to some patients than to others. This creates a tension between considering the wider context and the individual patient – trying to resolve this tension has become everyday work for GPs. This book is designed to provide some guidance in relation to dealing with this.

GP activities and consultations do not take place in a vacuum; rather, they occur in the social context of the time, and in the social context of people's lives. This is clearly more important with respect to some consultations and situations than others, but it is rarely irrelevant. All are not equal – people's needs vary, sometimes throughout their lives, sometimes as a result of inherent disadvantage. And as this book will demonstrate, some are more disadvantaged than others.

GPs more than any other group of medical professionals see first hand the impact and effects of disadvantage. For example, the occurrence of a sudden and unexpected myocardial infarction requiring urgent stenting or bypass grafting is a significant, potentially life-changing event in anyone's life. It is however experienced differently by the 50-year-old man whose critical illness policy pays off his mortgage, takes care of immediate financial concerns, and whose employer will allow a graduated return to his desk job, than it is by the man of the same age who is considered unfit to return to his job as a publicly employed gardener and whose wife is unable to visit him in hospital because she is caring for their grandchild, the child of their drug-misusing daughter who visits occasionally and only to ask for money. The eventual impact on these two families of the same event will be very different.

The purpose of highlighting these differences is not to deny or lessen the impact of the illness on the first man and his family. Such an event is significant, and will be associated with significant anxieties that may need to be worked through with help from primary care professionals. However, the anxiety and stress surrounding a new diagnosis like this cannot be dealt with appropriately by a GP unless he or she has a good understanding of the patient's social circumstances, and, further, what that social context is likely to mean for the health and wellbeing of his or her patient. Good GPs understand social context, and are aware that the sociology of medicine is as important as the pathology. So while providing care equally to all at the point of need is the aim of the NHS, it is evident that in fact we are not all equal. Even within the same patho-clinical situation, the social context may make similar clinical scenarios work out differently in practice. It is therefore necessary to take account of the differences that exist between patients or families in order to treat them appropriately.

Individual general practices differ in how they witness disadvantage at first hand. Some practices are situated in areas of multiple socioeconomic deprivation, where disadvantage is the rule rather than the exception, and which presents its own organisational and workload challenges. Other practices care for large numbers of specific groups of patients who suffer from a particular type of disadvantage (and may indeed have been established to take account of such a disadvantage), for example practices that serve the homeless or prison populations. For most GPs, however, they will see particular patients with disadvantage among other patients, who are, by comparison, relatively advantaged. All practices will encounter patients who are more disadvantaged than others (for example those with learning disabilities or physical disabilities etc.). For all of us, therefore, understanding the challenges and issues presented by these patients is extremely important.

Health inequalities

There are significant differences in health and health outcomes depending on social position. These are well documented but need to be remembered in the context of a book considering social disadvantage. We know that health outcomes, both in relation to morbidity and mortality, are socially patterned, and are influenced by social determinants. The health of individuals largely depends on the social conditions in which they live and work, and in turn their health may determine where they live and work.

There is a considerable body of work documenting the evidence relating to the social determinants of health.[3] As social factors vary between societies, communities and individuals, so too do health outcomes. Consequently, when considering individuals and their lives, these factors need to be taken into account. A number of models exist to describe and explain the interaction between processes resulting in health inequalities, including the well-known model devised by Dahlgren and Whitehead[4] in the early 1990s (Figure 1.1). All of these models recognise the complexity of the issues involved and acknowledge that social factors combine positively or negatively to impact on health outcomes. Although these models consider health inequalities in different ways, all accept that important social factors and processes include:

1 Individual factors such as age, gender, ethnicity and class (sometimes referred to as social position)

2 General socioeconomic, cultural and environmental factors such as employment, living conditions, education, housing and health care

3 Social networks such as family and community

4 Specific exposure or lifestyle factors such as smoking, diet, physical activity and alcohol consumption.

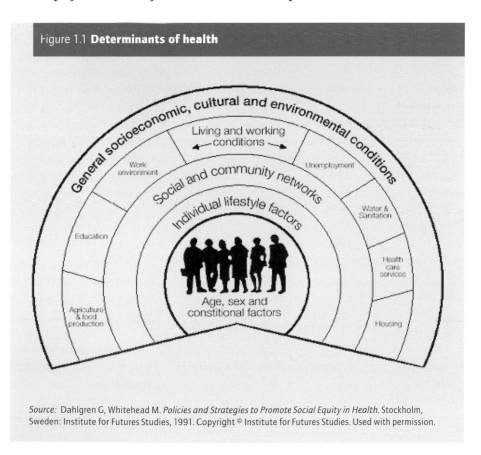

Figure 1.1 **Determinants of health**

Source: Dahlgren G, Whitehead M. *Policies and Strategies to Promote Social Equity in Health.* Stockholm, Sweden: Institute for Futures Studies, 1991. Copyright © Institute for Futures Studies. Used with permission.

Social processes make the coexistence of several of these factors more likely where one or two of them are present. For example, people living in poor housing who are unemployed may be less likely to exercise and more likely to smoke than those who are employed and living in good housing. The motivation and social support necessary to exercise or to stop smoking are also likely to be lower in those from more disadvantaged situations. Similarly, those with chronic ill health are more likely to be unemployed, outcomes that are both influenced by original social position.

In addition to the impact of social processes and structures, many social scientists argue the importance of life course on health and health outcomes. A life course perspective on health and its social determinants considers an individual's biological status as a marker of his or her past social position, and, as a result of the structured nature of social processes, as being liable to result in the accumulation of future advantage or disadvantage. So, disadvantage early in life is likely to accumulate additional disadvantage throughout life. Therefore, when GPs see patients in middle or old age, many of these processes will already be established. This life course approach can be applied to the study of health inequalities. This approach is an attempt to understand health inequalities from the accumulation and interaction of factors acting both early and later in life.

Life course factors begin before birth and will impact on child health. So, for example, poor nutrient supply to the fetus is likely to affect fetal development. This is a complex process, but it is likely that in well-nourished populations the interaction of diet with the mothers' pre-pregnancy nutritional status, metabolism and physiology will work to produce the best start in life. During infancy, the major risk factors are malnutrition and infection. Both are associated with poor social circumstances, and both can threaten survival as well as development. Childhood circumstances have particularly powerful effects on health outcomes, with some studies demonstrating long-term adverse health consequences. Disadvantage in childhood has been shown to impact not only on physical health, but also on cognitive and emotional development. More recent theories stress the role of the interaction between environmental factors and genetic predisposition, arguing that the physical, psychological and social environment may determine the way in which genes are expressed.

Thus, individuals enter adulthood with a health advantage or disadvantage relative to the rest of the population. There is evidence that where individuals can better their life experiences, for example by education and/or occupation, they improve their health outcomes. The worst health outcomes are seen in those whose social disadvantage continues into adulthood. Similar patterns are seen in ageing, with those from more disadvantaged groups experiencing ill health at an earlier age, and a more rapid decline in physical ability.

In summary therefore, the physical, psychological and social aspects of an individual are linked together very closely and need to be taken account of when we consider determinants of health, and when we consider the implications of disadvantage.

The implications of disadvantage for general practice

How then is disadvantage encountered in general practice, and what are the implications of this for GPs and for primary care teams?

Disadvantage may have many different implications, some of which are highlighted in the chapters of this book. However, the general implications of disadvantage for primary care are three-fold: 1) how disadvantage may impact on the way in which patients engage with practice, and on the particular expectations that they may have; 2) how disadvantage may create or impact on the actual problems that a patient presents with; and 3) how disadvantage may impact on the way that the practice has to conduct its interaction with that individual, group or patient population. Therefore general practices that find themselves situated in areas of multiple disadvantage are under unique and particular pressures. These have been documented particularly well in *General Practitioners at the Deep End*.[5]

In order for GPs to understand the implications of disadvantage, perhaps for an individual patient, they first of all need to understand difference, and the particular way or ways in which one patient might differ from others. This book gives help with this for a number of different groups that experience disadvantage. This will involve understanding the disadvantage itself as well as the particular impacts of that on health and the requirements for health care.

The effects of disadvantage, or, as we have already considered, multiple layers of disadvantage, are clearly seen in general practice in many ways. Some aspects of disadvantage relate to life course (for example older people) and some to personal characteristics, such as gender or ethnicity. Others still relate to the health implications of belonging to a particular group, such as the homeless. Within each of the core areas of general practice activity, differences between individuals can be relevant. Some areas where disadvantage may impact are considered below. We mention the relevance of literacy several times; primary care practitioners also need to be aware of the rather more complex idea of 'health literacy'. These overlap, and it is clear that disadvantage is associated with poorer health literacy.

Access to services

Accessing general practice is important for all patients, and obtaining an appointment with the preferred practitioner on a given day may be fraught with challenges. First, a patient needs to understand the system in his or her practice, which may differ from other practices. This may be explained in the practice leaflet, but it may not be readily accessible to all as it assumes a certain level of literacy. In most practices, a nego-tiation then needs to takes place with the practice receptionist. Even if these seemingly straightforward barriers are overcome, there may be additional physical barriers, for example for wheelchair users.

> Box 1.2 **Questions to consider for access**
>
> • Is 'access' to services built around patients' needs or practitioners' wishes?
> • How could barriers to access be minimised within your own practice?

Self-limiting illness

Self-limiting illness forms a considerable part of the workload of gen-eral practice. As models of working and options for reducing pressures within the NHS are considered in the context of an ageing population, this is one area in which more self-care by patients is regarded as eas-ing the burden on the health service. However, patients need to have the capacity to take this burden on themselves, they require appropriate literacy in order to read self-care materials, and they need to have the awareness and ability to access services when an assumed self-limiting illness continues. Such abilities include fairly complex emotional and cognitive processes. For some people, such as those described in this book, this may pose significant challenges.

> Box 1.3 **Questions to consider for self-limiting illness**
>
> • What models of care might be helpful in managing self-limiting illness in general practice?
> • How might appointment systems help with this?

Health improvement

Health improvement now forms a considerable aspect of the work of general practice. This includes screening activities, immunisation, anticipatory care and engaging with patients regarding behaviours that impact on health. All of these activities are more difficult in the context of disadvantage, where the idea of risk reduction may be an unfamiliar concept to patients. One of the fundamental responses to multiple disadvantage relates to low expectations with respect to medium- and long-term outcomes. Risk can be a difficult concept to convey to patients in any situation, particularly in relation to translating population risks to an individual patient. For patients whose expectation is that death before 70 is normal and to be expected, reducing cardiovascular risk may not be their main priority.

In addition, discussions about the behavioural influences on health are more complex than is often acknowledged. While it is true that several behavioural factors (such as diet, smoking, exercise, alcohol use) have profound influences on health, the political narrative in recent years regarding these has tended to emphasise individuals' responsibility for their behaviours, and therefore their health outcomes. This analysis results in the blaming of those who engage in these behaviours without seeking to understand the context of their lives, including that the particular pressures and situations they face may make correcting these behaviours very difficult. The most cited of these behavioural factors is smoking; this is understandable given the irrefutable links between smoking and several major causes of mortality. However, it is also true that smoking rates are highest among adults who have experienced disadvantage across their lives. Particular thought and care therefore need to be given to the ways in which we seek to engage with patients regarding such behaviours.

Box 1.4 **Questions to consider for risk**

- What are the different ways in which risk might be explained to patients?
- How could smoking cessation services be designed in order to meet the needs of disadvantaged people?

Management of long-term illness

Long-term illness management is a core part of the work of general practice. These activities present several challenges in the context of disadvantage. For several major illnesses (such as ischaemic heart disease, diabetes, stroke) long-term management is actually about risk reduction, a difficult concept to grasp, as discussed above. As part of this, dietary changes are likely to be recommended, but such changes will undoubtedly be harder to make for people with limited financial resources. Most long-term conditions require different degrees of self-care. As discussed above, this may be more challenging where disadvantage is involved, and more professional support is likely to be needed, which may require more contacts in primary care.

> **Box 1.5 Questions to consider for long-term illness**
>
> • What are the specific issues for people with Type 2 diabetes living in areas of multiple deprivation?
>
> • How might general practices adapt to meet the needs of patients with long-term conditions and learning disabilities?

Mental health

There are both general and specific mental health issues related to people experiencing disadvantage, and these are frequently seen in primary care. There are specific mental health disorders and issues for some groups, as discussed in later chapters. However, psychological distress related to the circumstances in which disadvantaged people find themselves is a common occurrence. The challenge for primary care is to diagnose depression where it exists, to engage with people in managing anxiety, and to identify those who either require or would benefit from referral to specialist services. GPs are often criticised for diagnosing and treating depression in people who are miserable because of the disadvantage in which they find themselves, but who are not clinically depressed. However, this narrative is more common among those not working with such groups; in reality differentiating between depression and misery is extremely difficult.

Box 1.6 **Questions to consider for mental health**

- How might a GP seek to differentiate between depression and misery resulting from social circumstances?
- What strategies can be used to assist such patients?

Vulnerable families

Disadvantage is often associated with vulnerability. Although the term 'vulnerable families' is most often used in the context of families with young children, it can also be aptly applied to older people. Dealing with vulnerable families in clinical practice requires a higher index of suspicion regarding presentations, and requires the use of safety netting. This adds to the complexity of consultations and interactions. Many issues for specific families that fall into this category are discussed throughout this book.

Box 1.7 **Questions to consider for vulnerable families**

- What is the role of GPs in managing vulnerable families?
- How are other professionals involved?

In summary, we have seen that there are some general and specific ways in which disadvantage manifests itself in general practice. This can impact on and affect all of the core activities of general practice. More time will be required to deal with these patients and families. Practices must not only be highly organised in order to meet demands, but also be able to be responsive to crises.

The ethics of delivering care to disadvantaged groups

The NHS was established so that all would receive the care that they need at the point of need, irrespective of their ability to pay. The ethical principle of distributive justice is about the fair distribution of healthcare resource irrespective of whether or not an individual can afford it, so that a person's right to health care does not depend on features of who they are, including their age, gender, ethnicity and socioeconomic status.

Consequently, disadvantage such as that described in this book should not impact on the health care that an individual receives.

The Inverse Care Law was first described by Julian Tudor Hart in 1971.[6] It states that 'the availability of good medical care tends to vary inversely with the need for it in the population served'. Evidence produced over the subsequent decades has demonstrated that this continues to be the case. As a result, many disadvantaged individuals may not be receiving the health care that they need. This is particularly true in areas of multiple deprivation where, although need is demonstrably greater, resources in terms of healthcare professionals tends to be much the same as in affluent areas.

Of particular challenge to healthcare planners is the paradox that policies which seek to deal with inequality may actually result in widening the inequalities gap, rather than reducing it. For example, if smoking cessation services are offered equally to all, they are more likely to be taken up by more affluent individuals and as such the better-off are more likely to benefit. The challenge for healthcare planners and providers is to consider the implication of disadvantage with regard to health improvement policies. The methods of engagement with more disadvantaged patients need to be considered and tested. This may include policies that discriminate in favour of disadvantage.

Linked to this is the important issue of resources. In the context of finite resources, rationing of care becomes a prerequisite of justice, so that resources can be appropriately applied to the services, people and conditions where most benefit can be achieved. In general, healthcare planners and politicians have tended to avoid doing this overtly, and it can be argued that those who suffer are those who are already living with disadvantage.

Role of general practice in working with disadvantaged groups

The principal role of general practice in working with disadvantaged groups is to deliver high-quality primary care to people irrespective of their circumstances. This includes ensuring multidisciplinary working, appropriate access to services, and designing services to suit the particular population being served, all of which are essential aspects of general practice.

However, it can be argued that general practice has an even greater role when dealing with disadvantage. It also involves a supportive role and an advocacy role; alternatively, this can be thought of as working with people and working for them.

Working with disadvantaged people

The process of working alongside people with different disadvantages may be challenging. It requires an understanding of the patient's particular circumstances as well as an understanding of any stigma to which the patient may be exposed as a result of disadvantage. This involves getting alongside patients with respect to the particular issues in their lives. For many disadvantaged groups this may provide an opportunity for professionals to attempt to raise their expectations in relation to the opportunities that they can expect for their lives. One example of a practical way in which primary care teams can help raise expectations is by identifying literacy issues.

Working for disadvantaged people

It can further be argued that the role of the GP does not merely include supportive functions, but may also include advocacy in so far as disadvantaged people are concerned. This may be on a personal basis as individual examples of the impacts of disadvantage arise. Advocacy also includes campaigning for particular groups, and in particular ensuring that sufficient resource is available to deliver care to disadvantaged groups.

Further reading

There are numerous texts on this subject. An excellent starting place is: Graham H. *Unequal Lives: health and socioeconomic inequalities*. Oxford: Oxford University Press, 2007.

- Department of Health. *Equity and Excellence: liberating the NHS* (white paper). London: DH, 2010.

- King's Fund. *Tackling Inequalities in General Practice*. London: TSO, 2010.

- RCGP Scotland Health Inequalities Short Life Working Group. *Time to Care: health inequalities, deprivation and general practice in Scotland*. Edinburgh: RCGP Scotland, 2010.

- Royal College of Physicians. *How Doctors Can Close the Gap: tackling the social determinants of health through culture change, advocacy and education*. London: RCP, 2010.

- UCL Institute of Health Equity. *Working for Health Equity: the role of health professionals*. London: UCL, 2013.

References

1. Duffy K. *Social Exclusion and Human Dignity in Europe. Background report for the proposed initiative by the Council of Europe*. Strasbourg: Council of Europe, 1995.

2. Rose G. *Strategy of Preventive Medicine*. Oxford: Oxford University Press, 1992.

3. Marmot M (Chairman). *Fair Society, Healthy Lives: strategic review of health inequalities in England post 2010*. London: Marmot Review, 2010.

4. Dahlgren G, Whitehead M. *Policies and Strategies to Promote Social Equity in Health*. Stockholm: Institute for Futures Studies, 1991.

5. Watt G. *General Practitioners at the Deep End: the experience and views of general practitioners working in the most severely deprived areas of Scotland* (Occasional Paper 89). London: RCGP, 2012.

6. Hart J T. The inverse care law. *Lancet* 1971; **297**: 405–12.

2 Sexual orientation and the health of transgendered people

Rafik Taibjee

Why this topic?

At times, this chapter is based on real experience as a GP and anecdotes as there is a lack of research in this area. I should warn also that the real-life scenarios may seem obvious but they *do* happen and have all been relayed to me in the last year. Some lesbian, gay, bisexual and trans* (LGBT) readers will disagree with parts of this chapter, and indeed LGBT people are a diverse group. [NB The term 'trans*' covers trans, transsexual, transgender and transgendered.] This chapter is not intended to reinforce stereotypes but instead to give the reader ideas of issues they might wish to explore with their patients. I used to say 'assume nothing' and you can't go wrong. However, this is not proactive enough for a group of patients who have such very specific needs, as I hope will be made clear by the end of this chapter. It is important to emphasise that the vast majority of LGBT patients are healthy and happy, and it is important not to assume they may be unhappy or unhealthy. Rather than listing facts as evidence of health inequalities, this chapter aims to give the reader tools on how to better serve this population, in need of better care.

> **Key learning points**
>
> - History, stigma and internalised homophobia can mean patients are reluctant to access health care.
>
> - Confidentiality is especially valued by patients.
>
> - There are definite lifestyle factors that make lesbian, gay and bisexual (LGB) patients in need of targeted health promotion.
>
> - Assume nothing when dealing with patients, but showing a little cultural knowledge can go a long way to encourage patients to open up to you.

Background

Until as recently as 1992, homosexuality was seen as a mental illness and was included in the DSM III classification and World Health Organization International Classification of Diseases, in various incarnations such as ego-dystonic homosexuality.[1] This may seem a long time ago, but to many lesbian, gay and bisexual (LGB) people this is a recent memory that leads to an ingrained distrust of the medical profession. To some, doctors represent part of the 'conservative' establishment and are more likely to be homophobic. LGB patients worry about being given a second-class service. Others feel that when they are ill doctors leap in and suggest HIV testing in a matter of seconds.

When combined with societal stigma, this exacerbates the problem, as did prejudices regarding HIV as a 'gay plague' in the 1980s. At the time of writing, it is illegal to have a gay male relationship in 78 countries out of 242, illegal to have a lesbian relationship in 45 countries, and there are seven countries with the death penalty for homosexuality, despite the United Nations Declaration in 2011.[2] It was as late as 1969 that homosexuality was decriminalised in the UK, and the age of consent was only levelled to 16 in 2001.

Stonewall is the UK's biggest LGB campaigning organisation. It was set up and named after the New York Stonewall riots of 1969. Its leaders believe that diversity is a notion best used to ensure that no one group is singled out in the equality agenda. It publishes the league table of good employers, and interestingly a few healthcare organisations feature in the top 100. To feature, an organisation needs to have clear recruitment procedures and an Equality and Diversity Group. The latter is consulted on policies that may affect patients or employees, along with Equality Impact Assessments before changes are made to an organisation. This would also fit with the NHS Equality Delivery System that is being rolled out across the NHS and which is supported by a toolkit.

With organisations such as Exodus, Homosexuals Anonymous and Evergreen International Inc. still existing, medical professionals need to be more positive with patients. Research through oral histories by former gay patients provides good evidence of the negative impact of the medical profession.[3] A significant minority of therapists in the UK will still attempt to help cure a patient of homosexuality and assist them in becoming heterosexual. As recently as 2013, some Christian organisations attempted to state that one can be cured and become ex-gay, in a London bus advertising campaign. This view is not based on any evidence.[4] *Cures*, a book by Martin Duberman, is one I would put on any doctor's reading list.[5] It accurately describes the experiences of men who as late as the 1980s were encouraged to suppress their naturally instinctive sexual orientation, and become straight. It outlines the at times gruesome methods used by the medical profession. I commend this book for highlighting how wrong we can be as a profession, even in an enlightened age, and how quickly opinion can shift. It also demonstrates how medicine and societal values are intertwined. For example, it would not be considered odd for a doctor in Pakistan to circumcise a male baby, or in India to use purgation as a form of Ayurvedic (traditional Hindu) treatment.

We live in a world that by no means fully accepts gay people. Combine this with the history of abuse from a conservative medical profession, and you can see why being 'out' to your doctor may feel difficult. Even the most confident 'out' people occasionally have to stop to check if it is okay to be 'out', and to what degree. That might be whether to hold hands with their partner in Iraq, attend a gay club or explain to a doctor that they are a 'bottom' (a receptive partner in anal sex).

Challenging discrimination

A lecturer at medical school only seven years ago included 'gay men sticking pepperpots up their behinds' as a cause of rectal bleeding. I remember my 'straight' friends looking around at me expecting me to challenge the lecturer. In fact, it took me a month to finally pluck up the courage to discuss this with him. I learnt where it can be hard to challenge people in authority even if they are wrong (and the doctor still is perceived by many as a figure of authority who has knowledge, which equates to power). I felt unsupported as none of my 'straight' friends challenged this obvious impropriety either.

Upholding anti-discrimination law is everyone's duty, and is included in the General Medical Council's (GMC) *Good Medical Practice* guidelines. Under the Equality Act 2010, there is a public sector duty. This makes it a requirement actively to promote the service to LGBT patients and to publish an annual report on how the organisation is performing in this regard, be it a surgery, Clinical Commissioning Group or NHS Board. There is also the Civil Partnership Act 2004, which requires all forms that ask about marriage to include civil partnership. In the UK a person can nominate anyone, including their unmarried partner, as their next of kin. And finally, in 2008, the Human Fertilisation and Embryology Act required that infertility treatment be granted to lesbian women in the same way as heterosexual couples.

Surely they'd tell me

Throughout their encounters with healthcare professionals, patients must decide whether it is important to tell their GP something. We make omissions of fact all the time, sometimes for brevity and at other times as they are 'personal'. LGB patients face this decision of internal censorship very frequently and in many everyday encounters.[6] Patients with less life experience will be less confident in knowing when a fact is important. Research consistently shows that only between a quarter and a half of gay and lesbian patients are 'out' to their GP. In the largest survey to date, of over 6000 people, it showed that 32% of gay men have not thought it relevant to discuss their sexual orientation, and in over half of cases 'the subject has not come up'. However, as you will see in this chapter, such information might be highly relevant to the care or advice they receive.[7] What efforts does your practice make to put patients more at ease about disclosing their sexual orientation? It is important also not to apologise for asking someone's sexual orientation or chosen gender role, as to do this further stigmatises the issue, and can put LGBT patients off.

Case scenario 1

A 20-year-old patient with dysuria has nitrites in his urine. The practice nurse sends off the urine for microscopy, which shows coliforms (a urinary tract infection). The patient is concerned about whether he should have told the nurse he was gay, and whether there is a relationship between having sex with men and urine infections.

It is worth noting the assumptions we make. While we nowadays would not assume, as in the past, that homosexuals are paedophiles, or are all effeminate, there are new assumptions pervading our culture: that gay men have lots of disposable income, are hedonists without responsibilities, are preoccupied by their physical appearance, are driven by sex and talk openly about it.[8]

Data management

Should telling your practice you are lesbian become a standard part of registration? How would your practice deal with this information? Would it be visible to all members of staff including receptionists, or on a separate clinical screen? These are difficult questions. Problems arise in communities where a receptionist knows the patient or their family well, and patients may not be entirely truthful if they fear disclosure or breach of confidentiality. However, without recording sexual orientation it may increase the number of times a clinician needs to start from scratch, asking each time the patient consults.

Another issue is one of definitions. Should one record sexual behaviour or sexual identity, or both? As you read earlier, knowing a man identifies as 'homosexual' or 'gay' is different from knowing he has sex with men. Black men, it is well known, often describe themselves as straight or bisexual even if exclusively having sex with men. How does one define bisexuality? Putting oneself into a particular descriptor can be challenging. Have you ever filled in ethnicity data? I'm a British-born man of Indian descent, whose parents were from East Africa. Am I a British Indian? I'm never too sure.

A new patient is registering and fills in an equal-opportunities monitoring form. He gets to the sexual orientation question, and goes up to the receptionist. He is clearly annoyed at being asked the question, emphasising he is straight, but wants to know why the information is being asked.

Consider what introductory text to give to patients before gathering equal-opportunities data so they can give informed consent to disclosing the information.

Monitoring

As Co-Chair of the Gay and Lesbian Association of Doctors and Dentists (GLADD), I have often heard members being concerned about being asked for their sexual orientation. Without at least starting on the road to gathering this data, we will never be able to demonstrate that organisations are free from discrimination or are spending resources fairly on this minority group. But on a personal basis we understand people's concerns. These concerns can be allayed by having a robust data management system and providing an explanation of what will happen to the information, and how it will be stored and used. How can you reassure patients? What is your practice policy? As an employer best practice is to monitor all strands of diversity. Even better is to provide opportunities for LGBT staff to meet and support each other.

A disgruntled patient writes a long letter of complaint about various things. He alleges he never gets an appointment because the receptionist hates gay people. How would you tackle this? How do you ensure you are treating patients fairly as a practice?

You are aware that gay men who have sex with men should be offered the hepatitis A & B vaccine. You want to search your computerised records to identify which patients to invite for immunisation.

Chaperones

There are also issues around chaperoning. In recent times it has become clearer that a chaperone should always be considered when undertaking any intimate examination of a patient. In the past they were generally only offered when a male doctor was examining a female patient. As a gay man I feel vulnerable when examining male patients too, especially when doing a rectal examination or feeling for a hernia, for example. In an ideal world one would have readily available chaperones all the time in a clinical setting, but the reality in most practices is somewhat different.

What policy is in place for chaperones in your GP practice? Does same-sex attraction feature in training of chaperones and clinicians? What gender should the chaperones be? What might a gay or lesbian patient prefer? Imagine how a lesbian doctor would feel having to ask for a chaperone for examining a female patient, thus potentially 'outing' herself to the patient and to the staff. Or, in the same scenario, when a patient says to a gay GP, 'You don't need one, doc. We're all men here.' How might you standardise practice?

Terminology

As with other groups, there is a sense of ownership of certain terms. In the USA in the 1970s, African Americans would object to being called negro or black, but often would describe themselves as such. Such self-determination is also the case for the gay community, who generally prefer not to be labelled with terms such as fag, the 'gays', queer, dyke, etc. If one does need to use a label it is better to use the expression LGB. For a while the group used to call itself LGBTQ, to include transgendered people, but both trans people and gay people, while wanting to support each other, may not have very much common ground, as one is about sexual identity and the other about sexuality. The 'Q' stood for either 'queer' or 'questioning', but is not used so much nowadays. The spirit of this should clearly be remembered because many people, especially adolescents, may be confused, and not yet wish to label themselves in any way.

So how many people are gay? Kinsey estimated through extrapolation that one in ten people are gay, but this is generally considered an overestimate, and represents having had a same-sex encounter. The current accepted percentage, used by the Department of Trade and Industry, of people who self-describe as being LGB is 5%,[9] one in 20 people, or at least one in every class in a school. The Office for National Statistics (ONS) says 480,000 (1%) consider themselves gay or lesbian, and 245,000 (0.5%) bisexual, but this was a Household Survey and only contained data for people 'out' to their families and friends.[10] It will be years before we truly know the answer, but interestingly the government used 6% when estimating the impact of introducing civil partnership legislation.

There have been some very interesting theories about paternal and maternal attachment, including Daryl Bem's theory,[11] but most gay people nowadays propose a deterministic view of sexuality being a result of several gene traits and the environment to which exposed during development. This is borne out by twin studies. Hence, you can understand that it is best to steer clear of the expression 'sexual preference' as this suggests volition or choice. Most LGB people would utterly refute and resent this because it gives fuel to the arguments of those who want to make gay people straight.

The other term to be careful of ignoring is 'bisexual'. This is a group of people who suffer discrimination from both the gay and straight communities alike, through a lack of understanding. One hears disparaging remarks on occasions and there is a fear that people who are bi may be more promiscuous, somehow needing to satisfy both urges, although this is something not borne out in fact. In the sexual health arena the phrase 'men who have sex with men' (MSM) is used. This is again to avoid labels, especially as it is known that black men in particular, even if exclusively having sex with men, do not call themselves gay and often describe themselves as bisexual.

> What terminology is used on your publicity and posters, and in the practice leaflet? Are you being as inclusive as possible, or could you be putting off those most in need? Stonewall has found that only 9% of lesbian patients recall seeing a non-discrimination policy and almost no lesbian images on waiting-room posters.

There is growing evidence that patients look at anti-discrimination policies. Having positive statements affirming that you value everyone can be very powerful. Displaying a rainbow flag (the gay six-colour variety) is also a good way of showing you are gay-friendly, for example by putting one on the glass of your door or by using a rainbow flag mouse-mat. And with Pride festivals and the International Day Against Homophobia (IDAHO) on 17 May, it is possible to have specific campaigns to reach out to your LGBT patients. But with knowing all this, my own practice had a heteronormative poster on display stating 'cigarettes make you less attractive to the opposite sex', so vigilance is important.

HIV

About 70% of all domestically acquired HIV infections occur as a consequence of sex between men.[12] I was asked by many gay colleagues when writing this to point out that just because someone is gay doesn't mean they have HIV (even in big cities it is more like one in ten gay men carrying the virus). Also you can get a better idea of a patient's risk by talking to them about their risk-taking behaviour. An example is a monogamous gay relationship with condoms, when compared with a straight couple using the pill for contraception.

HIV testing is needed if men are to know their HIV status. Yet uptake of testing among gay men is not high: community samples, such as a Glasgow study, suggest that up to 40% of gay men have never been tested, and only 30% had been tested in the last year.[13] The GP consultation is an important means of health promotion; however, more than half of gay men are certain that their GP does not know about their sexuality or (homo)sexual behaviour, and only a quarter have disclosed this information to staff at their primary care setting.

In my own research, I found that men in London and Birmingham would go to dark rooms (found in saunas or nightclubs). Those who were HIV positive would think no one would be 'silly' enough to come to a dark room and be HIV negative and have unprotected sexual intercourse (UPSI). Conversely, HIV negative men believed no one would be selfish enough to come to a dark room and infect people with HIV. Clearly this poor estimation of risk is a factor that needs to be addressed. Other reasons for use cited by patients include 'Sex is more exciting without a condom', 'I want to show him he is special' or 'I've already slipped up once so why bother now?'

It is amazing how many men still do not know about seroconversion illnesses, and also about post-exposure prophylaxis, which can be requested after having UPSI. This is clearly something healthcare professionals need to address when talking to MSM, and also when discussing risk behaviour if going to places like Amsterdam or Bangkok.

Over the last 20 years many charities have given out condoms, and these were usually extra-strong. There is no evidence for their use above standard condoms, and the need to purchase/obtain extra-strong condoms has been cited as a reason not to wear a condom at all. It might be worth discussing this with your patient also.

....

Case scenario 2

A patient has tested positive for HIV after a new-patient routine screening test. How might he be feeling? Stupid as a gay man who knew the risks? Worried what his friends will say? How will he tell his partner? Liberated as he may falsely think he can now have unprotected sex without fear?

....

Other infections

Human papilloma virus (HPV) was twice as common among HIV positive gay men as among HIV negative gay men, suggesting they may be at increased risk of anal cancer.

There has also been a worrying increase in syphilis in the gay population. An area of need often missed in general practice is oral gonococcus; here, a cause of infection is forgotten for sore throats and discharge in men, who can also be carriers.

Due to the nature of the sex, gay men are at significantly increased risk of hepatitis A, B and C. It is important that gay men are offered immunisation due to the risks of faeco-oral and anally blood-based transmission. Once again, knowledge of your patients' sexual orientation is required to do this. Unfortunately, in 2007, 28% of gay men responding to the annual sex survey reported having been vaccinated against hepatitis A, and 46% against hepatitis B.[14] Hence combined vaccines have not reached these at-risk patients.

Bailey's research shows that trichomoniasis, genital herpes and genital warts have been diagnosed in women with no sexual history with men.[15] Although gonorrhoea and Chlamydia are infrequently found in lesbians, bacterial vaginosis (BV) occurred more commonly among lesbians than heterosexual women. BV was associated with a larger number of female sexual partners and with smoking, but not with sex with men. These findings suggest that BV may be sexually transmitted between women.

Talking sex

A brief diversion to discuss this is important because knowing a little vocabulary can really give you some credibility with your patients. The first thing to say is that it is thought that only about half of gay men have anal sex regularly. So if a man says he is gay, do not assume anything. Those who do have anal sex tend to describe themselves as a 'top' (insertive partner), 'bottom' (receptive partner) or versatile (happy being either).

Because of this diversity of role, it is worth discussing 'compatibility' with the patient, as there may be an unmet need for psychosexual counselling or support with being intimate with partners. Also, erectile dysfunction needs to be discussed as well as anything the patient may have done to help with his condition. In clinical practice psychosexual doctors see gay men who can become so in fear of HIV that they stop themselves having types of sex that might come naturally to them.

Cruising is sex outdoors in public areas, for example in well-known areas such as Clapham Common. Cottaging is similar but uses public toilets as a sex venue, sometimes through glory holes (holes between cubicles). Both these activities are less common since it has become easier to be 'out' and also since the advent of the internet. Smart phone apps such as Grindr are now commonly used to locate nearby sexual partners. The 3 As of anonymity, affordability and accessibility have led to much more ease getting sex, which in turn has led to an increase in hypersexuality disorders.

The gay scene only serves a subset of the population you may wish to be reaching out to. Many gay men do not feel they belong to a gay scene and prefer to interact with a wider spectrum of people, or perhaps do not like the alcohol or at times sexually charged atmosphere.

Mental health

The majority of LGBT people do not have any mental health problems but it is known they are at more risk than the general population. Clearly happiness at work is important for wellbeing yet it is known that gay men are significantly more likely to have been unfairly dismissed or been bullied at work. It is also known that lesbian women report more verbal abuse than their straight counterparts, and research by Meyer shows this is positively associated with more deliberate self-harm.[16]

Gay men are over five times more likely to have engaged in deliberate self-harm (DSH) than their straight counterparts.[17] The Scottish wellbeing study found bisexual people to engage in DSH more than gay men or lesbian women. Although the evidence is weak, it would seem reasonable as it is well known that they drink more alcohol, and from a younger age, than their straight counterparts.

Gay people do live in fear, unable to visit places of the world in safety, or even hold hands in areas of London, with recent murders in Shoreditch and even Trafalgar Square demonstrating this fact. A large-scale study commissioned by the police in the UK found that one in five lesbian and gay people had experienced a homophobic hate crime in the previous three years and three in four of those did not report the crime to the police. Half of school children have been bullied when 'out' at school, prompting the 'It Gets Better' campaign.[18]

One-third of gay men, a quarter of bisexual men and over 40% of lesbians reported negative or mixed reactions from mental health professionals when they disclosed their sexual orientation, according to a survey conducted by Prof. King on behalf of Mind.[19] These reactions may range from a lack of empathy about sexual orientation to incidents of homophobia.

It can be difficult for healthcare professionals to get the balance right. In some of the accounts reported by King, mental health professionals were regarded as insensitive if they placed too much emphasis on sexual orientation in the clinical setting, while others were regarded as insensitive if they ignored it. Research by Stonewall emphasises the importance of acknowledging someone if they 'come out to you' even if to you it is not important or relevant.[20] Continuity of care is similarly important. Imagine if every time you visited your doctor's surgery you had to see a different doctor and each time decide whether to bring up your sexual orientation or not.

No mention of mental health should ignore the impact of 'coming out' on parents, friends and family. Parents may feel socially isolated, not being able to talk to their friends or even partners due to perceived stigma. They may also blame themselves. Signposting to resources is important. There are many groups around the world to support parents and family under the umbrella of Parents, Friends (and family) of Lesbians and Gays (PFLAG). On its website you can find resources useful to both loved ones and to the patients struggling to 'come out' to them. Learning how others before you dealt with things is invaluable. Here is how one mother described her experience of hearing from her 17-year-old son that he was gay:

> I didn't know anyone who was gay as far as I was aware. I drank too much. I drank too much and called my son, telling him all his achievements in life were worth nothing to me and I was no longer proud to call him my son. I was so selfish. I wasn't thinking about what it was like for my sons. But I look at them now with pride as they are two extremely well-adjusted young men – and I would not change them for all the world.

....

Rob had been seen in psychiatry outpatient departments for about four years, by about five different junior doctors. He had uncomplicated depression but never seemed to be improving. I saw him and he referred to his partner Alex at one point. I had to interrupt and clarify if Alex was a man or woman. He smiled and said I was the first person to ask him that and, after a moment of trepidation, he said he was a man. I asked him if this impacted on his mental health and this subsequently led to him explaining he was in a physically abusive relationship. Did I do the right thing?

Social isolation and internalised homophobia are amongst many reasons why LGBT people have a higher incidence of anxiety and depression. Knowing this, what services exist in your area to help them? Does the NHS provide any services like peer support groups or psychosexual counselling?

....

Bisexual people

Prejudice about bisexuality is called biphobia. It includes assumptions such as: bisexual people are 'really' either gay/lesbian or heterosexual;

they are confused; *genuine* bisexuals are attracted to men and women equally; or it is always a temporary *phase*. Work by King suggests that bisexual women are less likely than lesbians to report that their siblings are positive about their sexual orientation.[21] His research also shows that bisexual men and women are less likely than gay men and lesbians to have disclosed their sexual orientation to their GP.

Much research has focused on HIV/AIDS and has overlooked other aspects of bisexual people's health. There is evidence, mainly through Sigma research studies, that compared with exclusively homosexual men bisexually active men know less about STIs and have more unprotected sex with men.[22] This is perhaps due to finding it harder to obtain condoms and not accessing health promotion materials aimed at gay men. This would certainly apply to men who do not identify as bisexual, but who have casual sexual encounters with men. This is especially common for men of Afro-Caribbean ethnicity.[23]

Lesbian women – specific issues

Lesbians may have a slightly increased risk of breast cancer. This is thought to be due to being less likely to seek medical help, less likely to have children (or delay childbirth to later in their life), more likely to drink alcohol and more likely to be overweight than heterosexual women (hence also affecting cardiovascular disease).[24]

Perceptions of risk encourage women to participate in screening. Regarding cervical cancer, lesbians themselves believe they are at lower risk because of the disease's association with heterosexual sex. However, lesbians who have previously had sex with men (85% according to research by Bailey)[15] may be at some risk and there is evidence to suggest that women who have only had sex with women have developed cervical abnormalities, sometimes not HPV related.[24] In addition, smoking is a risk factor for cervical cancer that may increase lesbians' susceptibility even further. Yet lesbians are much less likely to be told they are at risk for cervical cancer than heterosexual women; some lesbians even report being refused smear tests. Healthcare professionals need to encourage all women to have smears, and to tackle this false health belief that lesbian women do not need a smear.

Reproductive health

There are increasing numbers of lesbians who are choosing to begin a pregnancy within a same-sex relationship. Lesbian women may choose to become pregnant in two ways: informally through their social networks, or through a fertility clinic.

The Human Fertilisation and Embryology Act 1990 retains the duty on clinics to take account of the welfare of the child in providing fertility treatment, but removes the reference to the 'need for a father'. Civil partners or same-sex couples can also be regarded as legal parents following fertility treatment provided that a Parental Responsibility Order is taken out.

Lesbians may seek advice from NHS professionals about having a child, for example through donor insemination. Comprehensive information about clinics providing this is available on the website of the Human Fertilisation and Embryology Authority (www.hfea.gov.uk).

Pregnancy brings lesbians into contact with a range of health professionals. Antenatal parent education is often cited as the most negative aspect of care received by lesbians. Health professionals often exclude the non-biological birth mother from discussions, but the recent changes in the law on legal parenthood following assisted conception should help to make care more inclusive.

Gay men – specific issues

The Annual Gay Men's Sex Survey has repeatedly shown gay men have specific concerns about how their sexual orientation is recorded in patient notes and who will have access to this information (e.g. will insurance companies charge higher premiums due to their risk of HIV? etc.).

Gay men have reported finding it difficult seeing urologists in particular due to a possible assumption of a female partner but also a lack of experience in managing any subsequent sexually related dysfunction relating to their illness, which may be different in gay men.[25]

Anal cancer is 20 times more common in gay men than in the general population. Anal cancer is associated with a history of anal-receptive sexual behaviour and with genital warts, HPV, hepatitis B, HIV, herpes simplex virus and being a current smoker. The incidence of anal cancer among MSM has continued to increase since the introduction of highly active antiretroviral therapy (HAART), and clearly more research is needed. The advent of the HPV vaccines has meant that this may have a significant impact on gay men. Although at the time of writing Health Protection Agency research is pending, one ought at least to consider offering private vaccination to at-risk men, as is being done in other countries.

Genital warts can cause a significant amount of distress to gay men. Knowing that there are vaccines that can help prevent not only genital warts but also anal cancer, there are growing lobbies for boys to be given the HPV vaccine as well as girls.

Adolescents

There are reports that some healthcare professionals have informed parents about a young person's sexual orientation without their consent. If a young LGB person's first experience with healthcare professionals is not positive, it may discourage future engagement with services in adult life. Young LGB people may have concerns about confidentiality, and it is important to anticipate this when providing services. Adolescents frequently report assumptions being made about their sexual orientation. This partly stems from sex education in schools focusing on heterosexual sex and contraception.

Case scenario 3

A 17-year-old girl came in asking for a repeat of 'the pill'. Performing the routine blood pressure check the doctor starts going through the missed-pill rules to ensure the patient understands when she is and isn't protected. Imagine how you'd feel if you were a lesbian who was only on the pill to help treat her acne.

Eating disorders seem to be overrepresented. In the Stonewall 2008 survey 10% of women reported having had bulimia and 7% anorexia. There is not much research into this area but specialists feel that male patients with anorexia are much more likely to be gay.

Growing old

How many times has a doctor visited an elderly man in a nursing home and considered the man's sexual orientation? Would the patient fit in? Have they been moved from the few friends who understood them and what it meant to have a gay identity? This issue is actually all the more important to LGBT people who are less likely to have family to look after them in their old age. As a trans* person, how might you feel if being washed by a carer? We also tend slightly to regard older people as asexual, but of course they may be very sexually active. Further resources and personal insights can be found on the Age UK website (www.ageuk.org.uk/).

Mental health

Many young people know they are lesbian, gay or bisexual by the age of 11 or at least know they are 'different', but may take another seven years to 'come out'. This period, often called the isolation years, is when they can be most vulnerable and in need of support.

Anyone under the age of 25 is at higher risk of suicide but gay men seem particularly at risk, perhaps exacerbated by actual or perceived rejection by their families. In comparison with their heterosexual counterparts, Fergusson's research from 1999 showed young LGB people are four times more likely to suffer major depression and three times more likely to be assessed with generalised anxiety disorder.[26] Young gay men are also seven times more likely to have attempted suicide than their straight counterparts. Recent Danish research has demonstrated that gay men in civil partnership are eight times more likely to complete suicide than married straight men.[27] Given this data, clearly any young person who attends with a possible psychological problem needs to be given the opportunity to discuss sexual orientation. Startling research by Stonewall in 2008 found that 50% of lesbians under the age of 20 reported deliberate self-harm.[20]

Research has shown that suicide risk is associated with identifying as gay at a younger age; not 'coming out'; not fitting with gender stereotypes; conflict with parents about sexual orientation, especially being told 'it is just a phase'; leaving home at a younger age; recent bullying or physical attacks.

Healthy lifestyles

In comparison with young heterosexual women, lesbian and bisexual girls are ten times more likely to smoke and twice as likely to drink alcohol in a given month based on US research by D'Augelli.[28] Furthermore, according to NHS Briefings, lesbian and bisexual teenagers are one and a half times more likely to have engaged in binge drinking in the past year, and are three times more likely to have drunk alcohol by the age of 12. Gay men are also less likely to look after themselves. Only 17% report eating five pieces of fruit or vegetables per day compared with 30% of the general population.[7]

Illicit drugs (e.g. methamphetamine) may be an increased risk for some young gay and bisexual men, particularly 'crystal meth', mephedrone, gammahydroxybutyrate (GHB) or 'liquid ecstasy' and its precursor gammabutyrolactone (GBL). These drugs produce euphoria but have sedative and anaesthetic effects. Usually sold as a slightly salty, odourless liquid in 30 ml quantities, less than 5 ml is usually enough to produce an effect, which can last up to seven hours. GHB has caused comas where patients suddenly wake up some hours later with no recollection of events, and is used as a rape drug. It is addictive, with extreme anxiety, sweats and shakes seen on withdrawal. There is also a significant minority of gay men who use these drugs to have 'chem sex', and a few who in fact cannot have sex without them. Some of these men may be HIV positive and it is well known that during weekends they may not take their medication, further increasing risk of transmission of infectious disease. Antidote, an LGB drug service in Soho, London, saw 85% of its cases being these newer drugs in 2012 compared with 3.2% in 2005, showing the need for doctors to have more training in dealing with these drugs. There are definite health disparities, with lesbian and bisexual women being five times more likely to have taken drugs, and three times more likely to have used cocaine (one in ten) or suffer from addiction (one in three).[28]

There are several gay magazines with a national and online readership. The most readily available include *Diva*, *Attitude*, *Gay Times* (GT) and the *Pink Paper*, which are accessed even by people who aren't 'out', and there are also free magazines such as *Boyz*, *QX* and *g3* that are available in bars.

....

Have you considered advertising services or offering health promotion using website banners or through the press?

....

Transgendered people

The issues faced by transgendered and transsexual people warrant a chapter in themselves. The prejudice and lack of acceptance that trans* people face limits their employment opportunities (despite legislation), their personal relationships, their access to goods, services and housing, their health and access to care, and their personal safety.

Terminology can be confusing and awkward. Is the patient someone who is transgendered, transsexual, a transvestite or just trans? It is best to dichotomise people who cross-dress and are transvestites from those who live the majority of their lives in their preferred gender role. This may involve hormones or surgery, but need not always. A term used in medicine is gender dysphoria: an extreme discomfort with the social role and phenotypic body originally born with.[29] Using terms such as gender identity disorder should be avoided as these sound judgemental. Just as with gay people, suggesting there is a choice or preference can be quite upsetting, and can make the patient feel not fully accepted for who they are. Data are very difficult to rely on. There would appear to be approximately 6000 people who have transitioned in the UK. In 2008 there were 2080 people with gender recognition certificates, 10,000 patients receiving NHS care, and about 1200 referrals.[30] However, the numbers of referrals seem to be growing by about 12% per annum, perhaps due to social or legislative changes.[31] A common pitfall is also to see gender as a binary entity. Many people are born intersex, or do not see themselves in one gender role or the other. It is important not to ask questions like 'Do you see yourself as a man or a woman?' and instead ask open questions like 'How do you see yourself?'

Surgery is often thought of by the medical profession as what trans people desire, but in fact only one-third of female-to-male (FTM) people have surgery, and that is usually mastectomy rather than phalloplasty (creation of a penis). The ratio of FTM to male-to-female (MTF) is 1:4. Yet there is a disproportionate focus of conversation on this, and some patients on reflection feel they were subject to unnecessary intimate examination by their doctor.[32]

To get gender reassignment surgery is still very difficult on the NHS. There is a shortage of resources and practice in this area can be open to challenge, as one of the leading authorities found when it did not follow GMC guidance. The rules are known as the Charing Cross rules, which involve living in the role for two years. These are based on the internationally recognised Harry Benjamin guidelines.[33]

Activists would say this is like saying someone with a facial scar has to wait two years before being offered plastic surgery. Rules and waiting lists are such that many patients turn to the private sector. A review of 80 qualitatively different case studies over 30 years demonstrated that the treatment is effective, and surveys suggest satisfaction with surgery of between 91 and 99%, suggesting that treatment is well received when it is obtained.[34]

In the past resources were so tight that it became a common belief in the trans community that to be prioritised you needed to be suicidal. The UK's largest survey of trans people (n=872) found that 34% (more than one in three) of adult trans people have attempted suicide. Similar rates were reported in a US study. Also research suggests that, due to the difficult process, some patients force themselves through it despite having significant concerns or doubts, presenting a front for the doctors' benefit.[32]

This in fact ignores one of the biggest barriers – the primary healthcare team. In a survey of trans people by Press for Change it was found that:

- 17% were refused (non-trans related) healthcare treatment by a doctor or a nurse because they did not approve of gender reassignment

- 29% said that being trans adversely affected the way they were treated by healthcare professionals

- 21% of GPs did not appear to want to help or refused to help with treatment.

The survey also found that little improvement had been made in funding gender recognition treatments and in waiting times over the past 15 years, despite significant legal changes and recent guidelines on commissioning services from the Parliamentary Forum on Transsexualism.[35]

Assuming that the individual does go through all the hurdles and successfully transitions, there are then issues the health profession needs to give better consideration to. Below is a list of common pitfalls:

- mental health problems can be misattributed to being due to being trans*, but clearly as people they can suffer exactly the same mental illnesses as others[32]

- FTM trans men are rarely included in breast screening programmes

- MTF trans women are rarely offered prostate screening

- intersex women report being repeatedly asked about their last period and their contraceptive use, while some are given smears (although they do not have a cervix)

- healthcare professionals asking for their 'real' name or failing to use the name and title that the person who is transitioning/has transitioned deems correct (e.g. Mr, Mrs, Miss or Ms).

Patients can be referred to specialist clinics but may also request the support of endocrinologists, psychologists and surgeons independently to help with particular aspects of their care.

The law

The Gender Recognition Act 2004 enables trans people to apply for 'gender recognition' and obtain a new birth certificate. In order to qualify, a trans person requires a diagnosis of gender dysphoria, *and* have lived in their acquired gender role for two years, *and* intend to do so forever more. Once certificated, trans people must be treated as of their new gender (sex) for all legal purposes, including health and social care.

Section 22 of the Gender Recognition Act 2004 makes it a crime for any individual who has obtained information in an official capacity to divulge that a person has a gender recognition certificate, i.e. is a trans person, or do anything that would make such a disclosure. This includes social and healthcare agencies.

The Sex Discrimination Act 1975, as amended in 1999, protects transsexual people, either intending to undergo gender reassignment, currently transitioning or previously transitioned, from discrimination in employment and vocational training.

In 1999 the Court of Appeal held that gender identity dysphoria is an illness under the National Health Service Act 1977, and that surgery is an appropriate treatment and as such it is unlawful for Primary Care Organisations to offer blanket refusal of funding for treatments in such cases.[35]

....

Case scenario 4

Andy, a newly registered FTM patient at your surgery needs the toilet, and asks the receptionist where the toilets are. The receptionist directs him to the disabled user toilets. How would you feel if you were him? Which toilets ought Andy to use? How would you deal with a patient who informally expressed objection to Andy using the same toilets they were using?

A doctor objects to prescribing hormone treatments for a trans patient as they feel this is against their religion. Is this permissible? What would you do if you were the senior partner or practice manager?

....

Concluding points

- Whether there is discrimination or not, clearly it is important to gain the confidence of patients so that they are able to disclose their concerns without any fear of judgement.

- The Equality Act 2010 and Human Rights Act 1998 make some requirements that it would be worth reflecting on when looking at your own practice: publicity material and public statements in your practice.

- To provide better health care there is a need for more research into the health of the LGBT population.

- Analyse your own assumptions and continue to be a reflective learner.

- Challenge the misapprehensions of patients, especially regarding their risk of disease.

- Where appropriate, commission services that address areas of specific need such as mental health, sexual health, substance misuse and eating disorders.

Applied Knowledge Test (AKT) questions

1 Which of the following might benefit from the HPV vaccine?

a Gay men

b Lesbian women

c None of the above

d Both (**a**) and (**b**)

2 Which of the following statements is correct regarding chaperones?

a A female doctor examining a woman will not require a chaperone

b A male doctor examining a male patient does not need a chaperone

c Chaperones should be used for all intimate examinations where the patient consents

d The chaperone should ideally be the same gender as the patient

For the following three questions, which is the most likely diagnosis?

a Alcohol dependency

b Usage of amyl nitrate poppers

c Crystal meth usage

d Mechanical back pain

e Slipped disc

f Viral labyrinthitis

g Depression

h Kaposi's sarcoma

i Venous haemangioma

3 A 40-year-old gay man presents with a purple skin lesion on his left temple that he has had for about three years.

4 A 25-year-old man presents to A&E after collapsing in a nightclub. His blood pressure was 80/50 on arrival of the ambulance but quickly rose to 120/70 by the time he arrived at hospital.

5 A 23-year-old Indian lesbian woman attends with a two-month history of insidious-onset, dull low-back pain not related to exertion and not helped by NSAIDs or physiotherapy. She is in good shape and works as teacher.

....

Answers: **1 = d | 2 = c | 3 = i | 4 = b | 5 = g**

Useful resources

- Gay and Lesbian Association of Doctors and Dentists (GLADD), www.gladd.co.uk.
- Stonewall, www.stonewall.org.uk [has useful LGB posters to display].
- London Lesbian and Gay Switchboard, www.llgs.org.uk, 020 7837 7324.
- Turing Network, www.turingnetwork.org.uk [a directory of sources of support for the entire UK].
- Gay Men's Health Charity, www.gmfa.org.uk [with listing for numerous social resources for LGB people].
- Parents, Friends (and family) of Lesbian and Gays (PFLAG), www.pflag.org.uk.
- Press for Change, www.pfc.org.uk.
- Transgender Zone, www.transgenderzone.com.
- Gender Identity Research and Education Society (GIRES), www.gires.org.uk [a legislative and carers' resource].
- Beaumont Society, www.beaumontsociety.org.uk [help and support for trans people].
- The Lesbian and Gay Foundation, www.lgf.org.uk.
- Institute of Medicine of the National Academies. *The Health of Lesbian, Gay, Bisexual, and Transgender People: building a foundation for better understanding.* Washington, DC: NAS, 2011, www.iom.edu/Reports/2011/The-Health-of-Lesbian-Gay-Bisexual-and-Transgender-People. aspx [accessed July 2013].

Further reading

- Duberman M. *Cures: a gay man's odyssey.* Massachusetts: Westview Press, 2002.
- Department of Health. *Mental Health Issues within Lesbian, Gay and Bisexual (LGB) Communities* (Reducing Health Inequalities for LGBT, Briefing 9). London: DH, 2007.
- Meads C, Pennant M, McManus J, et al. *A Systematic Review of Lesbian, Gay, Bisexual and Transgender Health in the West Midlands Region of the UK Compared to Published UK Research.* Birmingham: University of Birmingham, 2009.
- Hunt R, Fish J. *Prescription for Change. Lesbian and bisexual women's health check 2008.* London: Stonewall/De Montfort University, 2008 [a survey of 6178 UK lesbians and bisexual women].

References

1. American Psychiatric Association. *Diagnostic and Statistical Manual of Mental Disorders* (rev. 3rd edn). Washington, DC: APA, 1987.

2. European Union Agency for Fundamental Rights. *Homophobia, Transphobia and Discrimination on Grounds of Sexual Orientation and Gender Identity – 2010 update*. Luxembourg: Publications Office of the European Union, 2010.

3. King M, Smith G, Bartlett A. Treatments of homosexuality in Britain since the 1950s – an oral history: the experience of patients. *British Medical Journal* 2004; **328(7437)**: 427.

4. Bartlett A, Smith G, King M. The response of mental health professionals to clients seeking help to change or redirect same-sex sexual orientation. *BMC Psychiatry* 2009; **9(1)**: 11.

5. Duberman M. *Cures: a gay man's odyssey*. Massachusetts: Westview Press, 2002.

6. Adams J, McCreanor T, Braun V. Doctoring New Zealand's gay men. *New Zealand Medical Journal* 2008; **121(1287)**: 11–20.

7. Stonewall. *Gay and Bisexual Men's Health Survey*. London: Stonewall, 2012.

8. Ahmad S, Bhugra D. Homophobia: an updated review of the literature. *Sexual and Relationship Therapy* 2010; **25(4)**: 447–55.

9. Campbell D. 3.6m people in Britain are gay – official. *Observer*. 11 December 2005.

10. Joloza T, Evans J, O'Brien R, *et al*. *Measuring Sexual Identity: an evaluation report*. London: Office for National Statistics, 2010.

11. Bem D. Exotic becomes erotic: A developmental theory of sexual orientation. *Psychological Review* 1996; **103(2)**: 320–35.

12. Health Protection Agency. HIV in the United Kingdom: 2010 report. *Health Protection Report* 2010; **4(47)**, www.hpa.org.uk/Publications/InfectiousDiseases/HIVAndSTIs/1011HIVUK 2010Report/ [accessed July 2013].

13. Williamson LM, Flowers P, Knussen C, *et al*. HIV testing trends among gay men in Scotland, UK (1996–2005): implications for HIV testing policies and prevention. *Sexually Transmitted Infections* 2009; **85**: 550–4.

14. Hickson F, Weatherburn P, Reid D, *et al*. *Testing Targets: findings of the United Kingdom Gay Men's Sex Survey 2007*. London: Sigma Research, 2007.

15. Bailey JV, Farquhar C, Owen C, *et al*. Sexually transmitted infections in women who have sex with women. *Sexually Transmitted Infections* 2004; **80**: 244–6.

16. Meyer I. Prejudice, social stress and mental health in lesbian, gay and bisexual populations: conceptual issues and research evidence. *Psychological Bulletin* 2003; **129(5)**: 674–97.

17. Skegg K, Nada-Raja S, Dickson N, *et al*. Sexual orientation and self-harm in men and women. *American Journal of Psychiatry* 2003; **160(3)**: 541–6.

18. Dick S. *Homophobic Hate Crime: the gay British crime survey*. London: Stonewall, 2008.

19. King M, McKeown E. *Mental Health and Social Wellbeing of Gay Men, Lesbians and Bisexuals in England and Wales*. London: MIND, 2003.

20. Hunt R, Fish J. *Prescription for Change: lesbian and bisexual women's health check*. London: Stonewall, 2008.

21. King M, Semlyen J, See Tai S, *et al.* A systematic review of mental disorders, suicide, and deliberate self-harm in lesbian, gay and bisexual people. *BMC Psychiatry* 2008; **8**: 70–87.

22. Devlin W, Keogh P, Nutland W, *et al. The Field Guide: applying Making it Count to health promotion activity with homosexually active men.* London: Terrence Higgins Trust/Sigma Research, 2003.

23. Dodds C, Hickson F, Weatherburn P, *et al. Bass Line 2007 Survey: assessing the sexual HIV prevention needs of African people in England.* London: Sigma, 2007.

24. Bailey J V, Kavanagh J, Owen C, *et al.* Lesbians and cervical screening. *British Journal of General Practice* 2000; **50**: 481–2.

25. Weatherburn P, Hickson F, Reid D, *et al. Multiple Chances: findings from the United Kingdom Gay Men's Sex Survey 2006.* London: Sigma Research, 2008.

26. Fergusson D, Horwood LJ, Beautrais AL. Is sexual orientation related to mental health problems and suicidality in young people? *Archives of General Psychiatry* 1999; **56(10)**: 876–80.

27. Mathy RM, Cochran SD, Olsen J, *et al.* The association between relationship markers of sexual orientation and suicide: Denmark, 1990–2001. *Social Psychiatry and Psychiatric Epidemiology* 2011; **46(2)**: 111–17.

28. D'Augelli A, Hershberger S. Lesbian, gay, and bisexual youth in community settings: personal challenges and mental health problems. *American Journal of Community Psychology* 1993; **21(4)**: 421–48.

29. Burns C. *Trans: a practical guide for the NHS.* London: DH, 2008.

30. Wilson P, Sharp C, Carr S. Prevalence of gender dysphoria in Scotland: a primary care study. *British Journal of General Practice* 1999; **49(449)**: 991–2.

31. Reed B, Rhodes S, Schofield P, *et al. Gender Variance: prevalence and trend.* Melverley: GIRES, 2008, www.gires.org.uk/assets/LGBTSummit/LGBThealthsummit2008.pdf [accessed July 13].

32. McNeil J, Bailey L, Ellis S, *et al. Trans Mental Health Study 2012.* Edinburgh: Scottish Transgender Alliance, www.scottishtrans.org/wp-content/uploads/2013/03/trans_mh_study.pdf [accessed July 2013].

33. Harry Benjamin International Gender Dysphoria Association. *Standards of Care for Gender Identity Disorders, Sixth Version.* Düsseldorf: Symposion Publishing, 2001.

34. Pfäfflin F, Junge A. *Sex Reassignment. 30 years international follow-up studies after sex reassignment surgery: a comprehensive review, 1961–1991.* Düsseldorf: Symposion Publishing, 1998.

35. Parliamentary Forum on Gender Identity. *Guidelines for Health Organisations Commissioning Treatment Services for Trans People.* Melverley: GIRES, 2009, www.gires.org.uk/assets/Medpro-Assets/parliamentary-guidelines.pdf [accessed July 2013].

3 Caring for people experiencing homelessness in primary care

Angela Jones

Aim

Our society tends to have a fairly stereotypical view of homelessness, based on the image of a typical street drinker or injecting drug user, asleep in a doorway. As clinicians, most of us have a limited understanding of the housing system in our country and find it hard to understand why homelessness seems to be such an intractable problem for some people. Yet the truth is that most of us could be just one or perhaps two bits of bad fortune away from being homeless ourselves. The aim of this chapter is therefore to demystify homelessness and to outline some simple ways in which a primary care clinician can make a real difference to the life and health of a person experiencing homelessness.

Key learning points

- Understand the different types of homelessness

- Be aware of the causes of homelessness and how primary care can contribute to homelessness prevention.

- Help patients experiencing homelessness to obtain practical assistance including working with other agencies.

- Understand the common causes of morbidity and mortality for people experiencing homelessness.

- Offer health care to people experiencing homelessness in different settings.

The GP curriculum and care of people experiencing homelessness

The GP curriculum does not mention homelessness specifically. However, the skills needed to help and treat a patient experiencing homelessness are the same as for any other patient, only perhaps more so, in that patients experiencing homelessness frequently present with a range of complex and interrelated health and social problems. The skilled generalist is therefore the ideal practitioner to manage such a patient as he or she will have competencies in the main domains: primary care management of disease, person-centred care, problem-solving skills and a comprehensive, community-oriented and holistic approach. Generalists will also be aware of the importance of their own context and attitudes in their ability to offer good care and of the importance of a critical, research-based approach to their work. Of these attributes, arguably the most important is the ability of the generalist to offer the homeless patient a real choice about which of the patient's many problems he or she wishes to address first. This is an approach that is strongly empowering and enabling at a time when the patient is likely to be feeling vulnerable and powerless.

Defining homelessness

First of all, we need to know what we are talking about when speaking about homelessness. Homelessness is defined and tackled differently across Europe and across the world. The Housing Act 1996 provides a legal definition for England and Wales. The act identifies a person as homeless if:

- there is no accommodation that he or she is entitled to occupy

- the person has accommodation but it is not reasonable for him or her to continue to occupy this accommodation

- furthermore, a person is considered to be 'threatened with homelessness' if it is likely that he or she will become homeless within 28 days (e.g. because of eviction due to rent or mortgage arrears).

'Entitlement' to occupy accommodation can be obvious if a person owns a property or has a tenancy agreement. However, it is less clear in the case of a grown-up child of parents where the relationship between them has broken down. Is the child entitled to be accommodated by the parents? Is a person who is staying on a friend's sofa homeless? Likewise, whether accommodation is 'unreasonable' owing to its poor condition or to overcrowding etc. may be a matter of subjective opinion and can give rise to disputes about whether a person is homeless or not.

The European Federation of National Organisations working with the Homeless (FEANTSA), a pan-European non-governmental organisation (NGO) representing groups working with people who are homeless, has developed the European Typology of Homelessness and housing exclusion (ETHOS)[1] (see Box 3.1). ETHOS is a more wide-ranging typology of homelessness covering the various different situations that could be defined as homelessness in the physical domain (having an adequate dwelling over which a person or his or her family can exercise exclusive possession), the social domain (being able to maintain privacy and exercise relation-

---

Box 3.1 The ETHOS typology

It is clear from this typology that there are far more ways of being homeless or in housing need than simply sleeping rough on the streets and it becomes less surprising that there is a long-running controversy about the numbers of homeless people. The government in England used to publish statistics about homelessness that related to two groups only: homeless families (i.e. persons with children living in temporary accommodation) and rough sleepers (i.e. the count of people found bedded down during the night of an official street count). These numbers were never claimed to be an absolute count but, because the methodology was consistent, could be claimed to represent the trend. There are moves under the coalition government to change the methodology for counting rough sleepers and to look at a more absolute count. However, although rough sleeping represents arguably the most severe and harmful manifestation of homelessness, NGOs such as Crisis claim that the true number of homeless people is far higher than the official government figures, with 'countless thousands' of so-called 'hidden homeless' people living in squats, with friends, in cars, in caravans or tents, or in B&Bs.[2]

Does the number of homeless people matter? The answer is yes, because in order to provide for the needs of homeless people an accurate needs assessment must be undertaken so that services can be appropriately commissioned. As a GP coming across a homeless person, or someone threatened with homelessness in your surgery, you will need to know what sort of needs homeless people may have and what sort of services provide for these needs in your area. First of all, it might be helpful to understand why people become homeless in the first place.

---

ships) and the legal domain (having a legal right of occupation, e.g. rental agreement, home ownership). The ETHOS typology delineates four main groups of homelessness: *roofless*, e.g. rough sleeping; *houseless*, e.g. hostel accommodation; *insecure*, e.g. squatting or staying with friends; and *inadequate*, e.g. caravan, overcrowding, unfit due to damp, ill repair, etc. (see Table 3.1, overleaf).

Pathways into homelessness

Whether a specific set of circumstances will result in homelessness for any one individual will depend on a range of factors relating to that person as an individual, his or her social relationships and the structural and institutional context of the country/area in which he or she lives. The risk factors and triggers for homelessness are summarised on Table 3.2 (on p. 44).

Table 3.1 **Definition of homeless**

Conceptual category	Operational category	Living situation	Generic definition
Roofless	People living rough	Public space or external space	Living in the streets or public spaces, without a shelter that can be defined as living quarters
	People in emergency accommodation	Night shelter	People with no usual place of residence who make use of overnight/low-threshold shelter
Houseless	People in accommodation for the homeless	Homeless hostel, temporary accommodation, transitional supported accommodation	Where the period of stay is intended to be short term
	People in a women's shelter	Women's shelter accommodation	Short-term stay in accommodation usually due to experience of domestic violence
	People in accommodation for immigrants	Reception centres, migrant workers' accommodation	Immigrants in reception or short-term accommodation due to their immigrant status
	People due to be released from institutions	Prisons/other penal institutions, medical institutions, children's homes	No housing available prior to release, staying longer than necessary because no housing, no housing identified
	People receiving longer-term support due to homelessness	Residential care for older homeless people, supported accommodation for formerly homeless people	Long-stay accommodation with care for formerly homeless people (defined as more than one year)
Insecure	People living in insecure accommodation	Temporarily with family or friends/no legal (sub)tenancy, illegal occupation, squatting	Living in conventional housing but no legal right to remain there
	People living under threat of eviction	Legal eviction order or repossession order	Where the landlord has an eviction order or the mortgagee has a repossession order
	People living under threat of violence	Police-recorded incidents	Where police action has to be taken to ensure safety of victims

Conceptual category	Operational category	Living situation	Generic definition
Inadequate	People living in temporary/ unconventional structures	Mobile homes/non-conventional buildings, temporary structures	Not intended as a place of residence, makeshift shelter, shack, shanty, 'bender', tent, semi-permanent hut or cabin
	People living in unfit housing	Occupied dwellings unfit for habitation	Defined as unfit by national legislation or regulation
	People living in extreme overcrowding	Highest national norm of overcrowding	Defined as exceeding national density standard for floor space or useable rooms

Source: adapted from European Federation of National Organisations working with the Homeless. ETHOS – European Typology of Homelessness and housing exclusion.[1]

Prevention of homelessness

As a GP, depending on where you work, you may not come across many patients who are currently experiencing homelessness. However, you will come across situations that could result in homelessness if preventive action is not taken. Crane *et al*. in their study of pathways into homelessness of older homeless people in England[4] showed that in many cases homelessness could have been prevented. Examples of scenarios were death of a relative or close friend leading to depression and/or failure to cope, the breakdown of a marital or co-habiting relationship, physical and/or mental health problems, housing benefit or rent arrears problems, and problems with tenants or neighbours. The common factor in most of the cases in this study was that the people involved had little or no personal support from anyone. They frequently did not ask for help or did not know that help might be available. Their situation was usually known to a professional but it was not realised or detected that urgent action was

> ### Box 3.2 **Causal areas of homelessness**
>
> It is clear from Table 3.2 (overleaf) that actual housing factors are only one of four causal areas for homelessness.[3] The issues of breakdown in personal relationships, of ill health and of leaving various forms of institutional care (armed forces, social care, psychiatric units, prison) are not only very prevalent but also are often interrelated in any one homeless individual. It follows therefore that the pathway out of homelessness is likely to require action by the individual, and by those helping him or her, across a range of different challenges.

Table 3.2 **Risk factors and triggers for homelessness**

Cause	Factor of vulnerability	Trigger
Structural	Economic processes (poverty, unemployment)	Rent or mortgage arrears
		Eviction from rented or own home
		Change of status, e.g. from 'asylum seeker' to 'leave to remain'
	Housing market processes	Loss of tied accommodation
		Change of place for job
	Social protection/welfare	New arrival
	Immigration/citizenship	Access to affordable housing and social protection blocked, e.g. new-accession EU citizens not entitled to benefits in UK
Institutional	Shortage of adequate mainstream services and lack of coordination between existing services to meet demand or care needs	Support breakdown or no adequate support in case of emerging need
	Allocation mechanisms	
	Institutional living such as child or foster care, prison, long stay in hospital	Discharge
		Loss of home after admission
	Admission/discharge procedures	
Relationship	Family status	Leaving family home
	Relationship situation (abusive parents or partner)	Domestic violence
	Relationship breakdown (death, divorce, separation)	Living alone
Personal	Disability, long-term illness, mental health problems	Illness episode
	Low educational attainment	Support breakdown or difficulty getting adequate support
	Addiction (alcohol, drugs, gambling)	Increased substance misuse
		Criminal behaviour/risky behaviour

Source: adapted from Busch-Geertsema V, Edgar W, O'Sullivan E, *et al. Homelessness and Homeless Policies in Europe: lessons from research.*[3]

necessary to prevent the person losing accommodation. Crane *et al.* suggest that, particularly in the case of older patients at risk of homelessness, their only contact with services is via primary care. The key is to have a high index of suspicion that a patient in difficult circumstances may be at risk of homelessness and to ask direct questions about how he or she is coping. The next vital step is to know how to refer for further help.

Services for homeless people

Table 3.3 summarises the type of service that might be available for people experiencing homelessness.

Table 3.3 **Types of services for homeless people**

Service	Example
Prevention services for households at immediate risk of homelessness	Services offering mediation in cases of domestic conflict, rent or mortgage arrears, debt crisis counselling, etc.
Emergency accommodation for roofless persons	Emergency/night shelters
Temporary accommodation for houseless persons	Hostels, supported or transitional housing, shelters for victims of domestic violence
Non residential services for homeless and formerly homeless persons	Outreach services, day centres, advice services, health services, mobile food services (soup kitchens), floating support for ex-homeless persons in permanent housing, education/training and employment services
Accommodation for other client groups that may be used by homeless persons	Hotels, B&B accommodation, specialist support and residential care services for people with drug, alcohol or mental health problems
Mainstream services for the general population that may be used by homeless people	Advice services, health and social care services, welfare payment services, employment, education and training services
Specialist support services for other client groups that may be accessed by homeless people	Psychiatric services, counselling and relationship services, drug detoxification and treatment centres, services for former offenders and vulnerable adults

Source: adapted from Busch-Geertsema V, Edgar W, O'Sullivan E, *et al. Homelessness and Homeless Policies in Europe: lessons from research.*[3]

Housing and homelessness prevention

As a primary care clinician it is helpful to have a working relationship with your local housing department and know how to refer a patient who is in housing need or threatened with homelessness. A patient who is homeless or in housing need will often approach you for 'a letter for the council'. Be aware that just running off some sort of letter is unlikely to help the patent and is more likely to cause frustration for all concerned. Most councils have specific officers and processes to deal with home- lessness and housing need. If they require information, they will usually have a *pro forma* or will write to you asking for specific information, which you may be willing to provide with the patent's consent. Flagging up with the council's housing department that a certain individual is at risk of homelessness and needs an urgent appointment to discuss his or her housing options is the most useful thing that you can do. This is usually most easily done by telephone. Councils have a duty to assist people who are homeless or threatened by homelessness by signposting them to emergency or temporary accommodation options. However, shocking as this may seem, they do not have a duty to provide all homeless people with accommodation on demand. They must decide if someone is in 'pri- ority need' and medical evidence may be required to make this decision. It is this part of the process where a primary care clinician's written input may be requested.

Emergency accommodation and hostels

In England, if a council is making enquiries about a homeless person's eligibility for housing, it will usually offer emergency accommodation for a few weeks until the enquires are completed. This accommodation is often in B&Bs or hotels, or in self-contained accommodation within houses of multiple occupation (HMOs) but usually with shared bath- rooms/cooking facilities. These can be challenging or depressing places to stay, and, especially if a homeless person has developed a social circle within the homeless community, he or she may be lonely or frightened and surprisingly less happy to be there than you would expect. At least if you are attacked or bullied on the streets or collapse from an overdose, you are often in plain sight and there is a chance that someone will come to your aid. This is less likely in emergency accommodation.

There are two main types of temporary accommodation available specifically to people who are experiencing homelessness:

- night shelters offering somewhere to sleep overnight, sometimes with evening meal and/or breakfast but no daytime accommodation

- hostels offering shared or single-room accommodation, usually with catering provided.

Both of these types of accommodation are usually 'direct access'; in other words, the person can approach the accommodation provider to apply for the accommodation without being referred from another agency. However, there may be application procedures, exclusion criteria (such as no drinking on the premises, or even no active drug or alcohol use at all in the case of so-called 'dry' hostels).

Furthermore, in the UK, as most of these organisations depend on housing benefit from the local authority (LA) to pay the rent for the client, there is a considerable amount of bureaucracy and form-filling necessary to obtain the accommodation. As many LAs now operate a 'local connection' policy, hostels may require referral or endorsement from a street outreach worker to satisfy the hostel that the person fulfils the LA's criteria for local connection and is therefore eligible to have his or her rent funded. Finally, housing benefit does not cover the cost of catering, and, as part of the agreement, residents may be required to pay for meals out of their other benefits. This is a frequent source of conflict and can lead to the accumulation of arrears and ultimately eviction, as some may prefer to buy cheaper food and spend their benefit on other things. However, the supply of nutritious food at regular times is viewed by many providers as an important part of the hostel's 'offer' and the provision of self-catering kitchens can be complex and even dangerous to people who have been living on the streets and are not used to cooking for themselves.

The other characteristic of hostels, and also many night shelters, is that they are usually run by NGOs, who provide allocated support staff (key workers) to help residents address their homelessness and the underlying issues. Key workers, like all professionals, vary a good deal. Many are highly experienced individuals, who may have a long acquaintance with certain homeless individuals, which gives them a unique insight. They will often be able to spot when a person's behaviour has changed or when they are physically unwell. Key workers can be approached to obtain background information or a history from a patient who is not well enough to give his or her own account. They can be an invaluable source of information and 'intelligence' when making your clinical assessment.

Other services

There may be arrangements of other services available to people experiencing homelessness, but the exact configuration varies from area to area. As a GP, it may be useful to find out what is available, so that you can direct your patient to an appropriate agency to help with his or her needs. Day centres offer a warm place to sit, drinks or meals and a range of other facilities such as washing machines, showers, lockers, etc. Many also have visiting staff from other agencies who offer help with housing, employment, alcohol or drug advice, either on an appointment or on a drop-in basis. Your homeless patient may be on probation, in which case he or she should have contact with a probation officer who may also be a source of information and support. In some cities, there is a bewildering range of venues that homeless people may attend to obtain various resources, such as sleeping bags, clothing, recently expired sandwiches and other food. The street outreach workers (whose contact details can be found by getting in touch with the LA housing department) are usually the best people to contact if you have a patient with a specific social need and you are unsure of how to help the patient to access it.

Making a clinical assessment

Table 3.4 **Potential physical health problems among people experiencing homelessness**

Respiratory	Upper respiratory tract infections, lower respiratory tract infections, influenza
	Chronic obstructive pulmonary disease (COPD)
	Tuberculosis (TB)
	Lung cancer
Gastrointestinal	Gastro-oesophageal reflux disease (GORD)
	Gastritis (alcohol or stress related)
	Upper gastrointestinal ulceration
	Diarrhoea due to infection/malabsorption/opioid withdrawal
	Liver disorders
	Hernia
	Cancer of oropharynx/oesophagus
Neurological	Seizures
	Peripheral neuropathy
Trauma	Assault
	Falls
	Burns
	Road traffic accident
Skin	Sunburn
	Frostbite
	Infestations
	Infections
	Dermatitis
	Psoriasis

Cardiovascular	Hypertension
	Ischaemic heart disease
	Drug-related ischaemic episodes
	Venous thromboembolism
Metabolic	Metabolic syndrome
	Pancreatic insufficiency
	Diabetes mellitus
	Vitamin deficiency disorders
Infectious disease	Blood-borne viruses
	TB
	Skin infections
	Insect-borne infections

As explained previously, people experiencing homelessness will usually have a range of problems and any clinical assessment that you make needs to be in the context of the complexity of their situation. It is important to be always aware that a person who is homeless has a very complicated life and has to expend a great deal of time and energy simply on survival, maintaining his or her personal safety, keeping all of his or her belongings together and finding enough to eat. Going to the doctor is not usually prioritised unless it is really important. As with any patient, the driver for seeking medical help may not be that straightforward and it is very important to elicit the ideas, concerns and expectations of a homeless patient early on in the consultation, so as to prevent missed communication and potential frustration for both doctor and patient.

We do not have any conclusive data on the causes of death of homeless people in the UK. Recent research by the University of Sheffield for Crisis[5] has shown an average age of death of a homeless person in England (which is not the same as their life expectancy) as 47, and this figure is remarkably similar for other developed countries and is about five years lower for the roofless rough sleepers. This research also showed that homeless people die of conditions that are generally thought of as treatable. Deaths from trauma and environmental conditions such as heat or cold, although higher than in the general population, are remarkably low in comparison with deaths due to illness. This means that, although homeless people are dying younger than the norm for their society, they are mostly dying of treatable illness such as COPD, ischaemic heart disease, liver disease, various malignancies, thrombotic disease and acute infections, and also of the consequences of addiction to alcohol and drugs. Most if not all of these are ambulatory care-sensitive conditions that are ideally managed in primary care. It follows that, when a homeless person presents to a doctor, we should be aware that this person is at risk of premature death from treatable causes and assess them accordingly.

It is also acknowledged that physical complaints often present at a more advanced stage in this group than in the general population, so it is vital that a full examination is undertaken to ensure that the extent of the clinical problem/problems is understood. Having said that, in a person known to have five different clinical problems (such as, for instance, alcohol dependence, previous perforation of peptic ulcer, bipolar disorder, hepatitis C and scabies), it may be best, on the first presentation with intolerable itching, to concentrate on the scabies while mentioning that it would be good to check out the liver at some point, in case it is contributing to the problem. The patient then has the choice of engaging in the discussion about the liver or returning at another date to do so. Empowering an otherwise un-empowered individual to choose which of their issues they wish to tackle first can be the beginning of a valuable and ongoing therapeutic relationship. Thus, although it can be a difficult balancing act between ensuring that serious illness is addressed and allowing the patient autonomy in the consultation, this is a task that a good generalist is ideally placed to undertake.

The other challenge in treating people who are homeless is that differential diagnosis for *common symptoms* needs to include not only the usual illnesses, but also may be skewed to presentations less commonly encountered in the general population. Here are some examples:

Presenting with cough

Viral infection is most likely. However, homeless patients are at greater risk of bacterial infection, presumably due to immunosuppression related to poor nutrition, environmental stress, exposure, co-infections, etc. *Remember TB*, which in many countries is very common in homeless, drug-using and prison populations.

Presenting with vomiting

In this population, vomiting is more commonly a symptom of chemical gastritis secondary to alcohol, or to alcohol or drug withdrawal, than a symptom of a viral infection. This group still get perforated peptic ulcers, which is rare in the usual population. *Beware of vomiting blood*. This is difficult to assess in this group because oesophageal varices are more common than in the general population, as are Mallory–Weiss tears.

Presenting with limb pain

The extent of vascular, especially venous, damage due to injecting drug use among homeless drug users can be horrific to behold, and limbs should always be fully examined to check for thrombotic complications. Femoral and axillary deep-vein thromboses (DVTs) are all too common, and are sometimes combined with infection. These are potentially life threatening or lead to long-term disability if not treated early and aggressively.

Presenting with itching

Homeless patients will usually assume that they have picked up an infestation when they develop itching. This is not always the case and consideration should be given to systemic reasons, such as liver disease, for itching. However, infestations of various kinds are more common in people experiencing homelessness than in the general population. Scabies is diagnosable by searching for the classical distribution of burrows between fingers or toes. It is important to explain and treat the ongoing allergic manifestation of scabies, which persists for several weeks after the insecticide treatment, in order to avoid unnecessary multiple treatments. Having said that, it is often necessary to give the advised second treatment at two weeks and reinfestation from untreated persons also occurs. Head lice are also common and diagnosable by inspecting the head or combing. Clothing lice are rarely found in the general population but do occur, particularly in rough sleepers or people who do not usually undress at night. The lice are visible along the seams of clothing and migrate off the clothing to bite almost anywhere, causing severe itching. Treatment is usually with malathion preparations. Clothing and sleeping bags need to be either replaced or washed and then tumble dried on a high setting to kill the lice. Many shelters/homeless hostels are familiar with what to do to avoid having to discard all the clothing.

Foot pain and mouth problems

Finally, people experiencing homelessness will present with problems outside the usual range of expertise for GPs such as foot pain and mouth problems. It pays to learn to perform a competent preliminary examination of feet and mouth, as your patient will have limited access to podiatry or dentistry. Also it helps to arm yourself with some sensible practical advice to offer regarding foot care and dental care. Data can be collected too, so that you can argue for commissioning of accessible dentistry and podiatry for the homeless population, if there is none available in your area. Be aware that people who are homeless are at high risk of oral and ENT malignancy due to the high rates of alcohol intake and almost universal incidence of tobacco smoking. Furthermore, peripheral neuropathy not unlike that in diabetes mellitus can occur in heavy drinkers, laying them open to similar risks of painless ulceration.

Mental ill health among people experiencing homelessness

It is generally acknowledged that people experiencing homelessness are far more likely to suffer from a mental illness and to have experienced adverse and damaging life events than the general population. Unpicking the relationship between homelessness and mental illness is not easy, in that people with mental health problems are more vulnerable to the type of life events and behaviours that can culminate in losing one's home. However, the state of homelessness is itself a potent trigger or cause for exacerbation of a range of mental health problems. Substance misuse is also very common among people who are homeless, involving particularly heroin, crack cocaine and alcohol, frequently with poly-drug use. This prevalence of substance misuse complicates the diagnosis and treatment of mental ill health, as many psychiatric services are unwilling to perform a mental health assessment on people who are actively using substances.

Responding to a homeless person in mental distress can be therefore very challenging. Our services are not well designed to cope with or to offer comfort and help to homeless people who are mentally unwell.[6] The principles of making a mental health assessment are the same as for any other patient and will require an in-depth examination of the patient's circumstances and life history. Family background and early years are often particularly illuminating, with a higher incidence of traumatic events, particularly in childhood, than in the general population. However, it may not be possible or sensible to explore all these factors while the person has no accommodation or place of safety and is very vulnerable. A more pragmatic problem-solving approach is often more effective when the patient is distressed, initially engaging with the practical issues such as food, clothing, benefits and shelter. Simultaneously, information can be gathered, an outline risk assessment made and follow-up arranged, for the following day if possible, or sooner if appropriate.

Some experience of psychiatry during postgraduate training, either in inpatient or liaison psychiatry, is not essential, but is definitely a benefit when working with people who are homeless, as it enhances your confidence in dealing with this kind of high-risk situation. It is vital, as a primary care physician treating homeless people, to develop supportive relationships with your local psychiatric services if at all possible. You will need help with assessment and management of complex cases, involving co-morbidity/forensic issues and often requiring some detective work to uncover previous psychiatric history. It may be worth pointing out that you can be helpful to the psychiatric services by avoiding admission and enabling management of these cases in the community, in return for their support and advice.

However, there will also be occasions when a homeless person will need to be deprived of liberty and compulsorily detained in order to perform the required assessment and/or establish the correct treatment for a suspected or known mental illness. The case for compulsory treatment may be clear in that the person has become a danger to others. Danger to self is a far more tricky concept, especially in the situation of long-term rough sleeping, where the homeless person has established that he or she can live for prolonged periods on the streets. The question of the extent of harm that this homeless condition itself is causing can be key to deciding if the person is a danger to him or herself. Psychiatric professionals who are unfamiliar with working with rough sleepers may be unwilling to compulsorily detain people with history of long-term rough sleeping, as the perception is that rough sleeping is the person's choice. Interestingly, in my experience, it is the more experienced homelessness professionals such as outreach workers who can pick out the rough sleeper who is not there from choice or expedience, but whose mental state is the key contributing factor to his or her homeless state. Visiting or at least contacting your patient on the psychiatric unit after compulsory detention is an important role for primary care professionals, in order to ensure that the staff understand the homelessness issues and to try to enable suitable discharge arrangements.

Special aspects of prescribing for people experiencing homelessness

It has to be acknowledged that medication is a difficult issue when you are homeless. Carrying medication is fraught with difficulty, as the drugs are liable to be lost or stolen or in some cases sold to raise money for other purposes. Certain prescription drugs are known to be diverted to use by substance misusers, taken by mouth or ground up and injected as an adjunct or substitute for street drugs (see Box 3.3, overleaf, for examples). Prescribing these drugs to any patient but especially to a vulnerable homeless person or to a person who is known or suspected to have an addiction problem is best avoided. Nutritional supplement drinks are popular, as they are often regarded as a substitute for food, allowing available funds to be diverted to other needs.

It is sensible to have a policy within the practice, which all clinicians are willing to adhere to, about how to respond to requests for these medications. This will avoid conflict and help clinicians to be prepared with consistent and sensible alternatives to offer to the patient. The policy could also include guidance about the length of prescriptions. For patient

> ### Box 3.3 **Commonly 'diverted' prescription drugs**
>
> - Codeine including when combined with paracetamol or non-steroidal anti-inflammatory drugs (NSAIDs).
> - Dihydrocodeine, tramadol, oxycodone and other opioids.
> - Benzodiazepines.
> - Z-drugs (e.g. zopiclone, zolpidem).
> - Procyclidine.
> - Sildenafil.
> - Cyclizine.
> - Nutritional supplements/sip feeds.
> - Gabapentin.
>
> NB This list is subject to change over time depending on local trends and 'fashions'.

safety reasons, it can be helpful to issue short prescriptions, thus reducing the amount of medication that has to be carried around. The most vulnerable persons on medications can benefit from daily prescription/daily pick-up. In most cases, this will mean issuing several serial one-day prescriptions, although in some jurisdictions arrangements are available for daily dispensing from a single prescription for certain medications.

Conclusion

I hope this chapter has served not only to inform you about the complexities of the world of homelessness but also to inspire you to engage with the next homeless patient you come across, with a certain confidence that you have some understanding of the patient's situation and what you may be able to offer. I also hope that you will be alert to the personal disaster that homelessness is and will be able to spot potential situations where, by judicious referral to appropriate support, you can prevent someone from becoming homeless. Ultimately, the most important thing you can offer is yourself – to approach the patient as a person who is experiencing homelessness, rather than one of 'the homeless'. In a recent radio broadcast, a contributor who had been homeless in the past was asked what the turning point had been for him, and he recalled that it was when the arresting officer at the police station said to him, 'Fancy a cup of tea, mate?' It was the first time in a very long time that someone had shown him a human kindness – and it was enough to turn his life around.

Further reading

- Wright N. *Homelessness: a primary care response*. London: RCGP, 2002.

References

1. European Federation of National Organisations working with the Homeless. ETHOS – European Typology of Homelessness and housing exclusion. 2007. www.feantsa.org/spip. php?article120 [accessed July 2013].

2. Reeve K. *The Hidden Truth about Homelessness: experiences of single homelessness in England*. London: Crisis, 2011, www.crisis.org.uk/data/files/publications/ HiddenTruthAboutHomelessness_web.pdf [accessed July 2013].

3. Busch-Geertsema V, Edgar W, O'Sullivan E, *et al. Homelessness and Homeless Policies in Europe: lessons from research*. Brussels: Feantsa, 2010, www.york.ac.uk/media/chp/documents/2010/ Homelessness%20and%20Homeless%20Policies%20in%20Europe.pdf [accessed July 2013].

4. Crane M, Warnes T, Fu R, *et al. Preventing Homelessness among Older People: lessons for practice*. Sheffield: Sheffield Institute for Studies on Ageing, n.d., www.shef.ac.uk/content/1/ c6/04/91/53/Manual1.pdf [accessed July 2013].

5. Thomas B. *Homelessness: a silent killer*. London: Crisis, 2011, www.crisis.org.uk/data/files/ publications/Homelessness%20-%20a%20silent%20killer.pdf [accessed July 2013].

6. Seager M. Homelessness is more than houselessness: a psychologically-minded approach to inclusion and rough sleeping. *Mental Health and Social Inclusion* 2011; **15 (4)**: 183–9.

4 Caring for Travelling communities in primary care

Nwakuru Nwaogwugwu, Joseph O'Neill and Paramjit Gill

Aim

This chapter aims to provide an overview of health, as experienced by Traveller communities. Unique aspects of their culture and beliefs will be considered with reference to the impact on health inequalities and provision of care.

Key learning points

- Appreciate that Traveller communities are made up of different groups with shared cultural origins.

- Consider an overview of the values, cultures and beliefs experienced by Traveller communities and how this affects healthcare access and provision.

- Understand the Traveller community's experience of health and social inequality, and how this impacts on healthcare access and provision.

- Be aware of the complexities, but importance, of a sensitive and holistic approach to care.

Travellers and Gypsies: a background

Traveller communities refer to a number of groups who share similar customs, such as living in close communities and Travelling, but who differ in their historical origins and cultural beliefs.[1,2] They include:

- Romany Gypsies
- Irish Travellers
- Scottish Gypsy Travellers
- Welsh Gypsies (Kale)
- Bargees or Boat Dwellers
- circus/fairground showmen – Travellers by occupation
- New Travellers – have opted for the Traveller lifestyle.

Here, the term Traveller communities, Travellers and Gypsies may be used synonymously, with reference made to specific groups when required. It is useful to note that Travellers may address non-Travellers as Gadze or other similar variants, Gaujo, Gorgio or Gorjer.[3]

It is difficult to determine the number of Gypsies and Travellers residing in the UK as they are poorly captured due to several factors:

1. The nomadic lifestyle of some Travellers makes it practically difficult to obtain the necessary data[4]

2. Travellers have previously not been recognised as a separate ethnic group in the census and so have simply not been counted.[1]

It is important to be aware that Romany Gypsies and Irish Travellers are recognised as ethnic minority groups according to the Race Relations Act 1976.[5] This act is a function of their ethnicity and not their Travelling status, and so applies to both mobile and settled Travellers alike. It recognises that 'less favourable' treatment towards this group by healthcare or other public bodies is discrimination.[5]

Estimates, from methods such as bi-annual caravan counts, number British Traveller populations in the region of 300,000, with Romany Gypsies and Irish Travellers making up the majority.[1,6] However, as the 2011 Census now includes Gypsies and Travellers as a separate ethnic group, they form 0.1% of the population of England and Wales.[7]

Romany Gypsies are thought to originate from Northern India, and over time have migrated across Asia, into Europe and the British Isles.[8] They have experienced a long history of discrimination and persecution including slavery and expulsion from several European countries, while being barred from entering others, including England, for a time.[8] In the seventeenth century, laws were enforced that restricted the practice of their culture – preventing the wearing of traditional dress, or speaking of Romani, or the gathering of Romany people.[8]

The origin of Irish Travellers is less clear, although one school of thought suggests they descend from peasants who were driven out from their land during the time of Cromwell's campaign or during the Great Famine.[3]

Marginalisation from society remains a current issue in Traveller communities[8,9] and the enduring influence of their previously negative experiences may explain why they remain suspicious, and at times distrusting, of the main society.

Travellers and Gypsies: health and social disparity

Studies of Traveller health and social demographics, although limited, unanimously describe a community with increased health burden and poor health outcomes in comparison with other ethnic minority groups, and with the general population.[8,10] This health inequality, in addition to difficulties accessing health services, especially primary care services, is referred to as a 'double disadvantage' by the Department of Health.[11]

There is also a disparity found socially and in education.[10,12] There are underlying contributory factors that are better understood by considering the social determinants of health [those environmental factors that affect health][13] in Traveller communities. These are further discussed in Chapter 1.

The living environments of Traveller communities are often insecure and poorly serviced.[6] Reliable accommodation is needed in order to access most public services, but opportunities to maintain businesses or access employment and education are likewise threatened if the 'environment' is unstable. This further contributes to their social exclusion and decline in socioeconomic status.[12]

The provision of stable living environments for Travelling communities is problematic as there is a shortage of authorised sites.[6] Approximately 50% of Travellers are thought to live in conventional, 'bricks and mortar' housing, with a quarter of those living illegally on unauthorised sites.[6] Unauthorised sites are usually located in undesirable areas such as by motorways, rubbish tips or sewage works, where access to basic amenities is likely to be poor, and standards of living well below that expected of social housing.[6] In addition, they face regular cycles of eviction.[6,12]

The decision to settle in conventional housing may often follow a period of recurrent evictions, inadequate provisions on a site or health or education concerns.[12] Unfortunately this may mean separation from a close network of friends and family. It may also mean that they experience racial discrimination and encounter some intolerant members in the local communities they move into,[12] somewhat reminiscent of their historical experiences.[8]

In the UK, pressures to start rebuilding after the Second World War meant that many publicly owned Traveller/caravan sites were used up.[14] New legislation in 1994 meant that Traveller communities were expected to secure and purchase their own land.[15] However, even when land was privately purchased, applications for planning permission caused, and still cause, tensions with local residents and communities.[4,12] Over the years grants have been allocated to local housing authorities for the purposes of purchasing and maintaining the upkeep of Traveller sites. However, access to and adequate use of these grants is variable across the country.[12]

The Department of Health 'inclusion health' document describes a socially excluded group as 'those people who are 1, Suffering multiple and enduring disadvantage and are 2, Cut off from the opportunities most of us take for granted'.[11] The Race Relations (Amendment) Act 2000 placed a statutory duty on public bodies, health care included, to 'eliminate unlawful racial discrimination and promote equality of opportunity' in recognised minority groups.[16] Despite this, Traveller communities still fit the 'socially excluded' criteria, and when the added influence of cultural beliefs and the impact of discrimination are considered, the complexities of tackling and managing health and social exclusion become apparent.

Efforts have been made nationally and internationally to address issues of social exclusion in Travelling communities and to consider their health status and beliefs.[3,9] The Decade of Roma Inclusion 2005–15 is an incentive initiated by several European governments, which aims to improve the socioeconomic status and promote the social inclusion of Romany Gypsies. The Decade recognised health, education, employment and housing as key areas that, if prioritised and worked upon, could result in improved overall Romany Gypsy welfare.[17]

The NHS Primary Care Service Framework (PCSF) describes a range of 'enhanced service provision specifications for PCT commissioners', and considers a holistic approach to the provision of care to various groups, Gypsies and Travellers being one of them.[1] Within this framework it suggests that access to and provision of healthcare services for Travelling communities should be of the same 'high quality' standard currently available to the general population.[1] It should also be accepted that the development of such programmes requires time, as well as good relationships and partnerships between health care and Travelling communities.[1]

MRCGP and the curriculum

Gypsy and Traveller health is reflected in all areas of the GP curriculum. However, in the context of health inequality, GPs should explore and demonstrate an understanding of the following curriculum statements.

Statement 2.01 The GP Consultation in Practice [18]

• Recognise that patients are diverse: that their behaviour and attitudes vary as individuals and with age, gender, ethnicity and social background, and that you should not discriminate against people because of those differences.

• Understand how the values and beliefs prevalent in the local culture impact on patient care.

- Understand how the demography and ethnic and cultural diversity of your practice population impact on the range and presentation of illness in the individual consultation.

Statement 2.04 Enhancing Professional Knowledge [19]

- Implement a community-based approach to disease prevention through effective multidisciplinary and interdisciplinary teamwork.

- Recognise the inequalities of healthcare delivery and how some evidence may not reflect the diverse nature of the population you are working with.

- Use clinical examples that reflect your experience of working in the community and the impact of disease on the individual and the family in the widest sense (physiological, psychological, social and cultural).

Statement 3.01 Healthy People: promoting health and preventing disease [20]

- Use routinely available data to describe the health of the patient's local population, compare it with that of other populations, and identify localities or groups with poor health within it.

- Engage in the implementation of locally agreed health programmes.

- Demonstrate tolerance and understanding of the patient's experiences, beliefs, values and expectations regarding preventive medicine such as screening and lifestyle modification.

The challenges in primary health care

In order to provide holistic care it is important to understand the underlying ethics, values, beliefs and cultures of both the patient and the GP, as well as the clinical and social aspects.[18] This fundamental understanding is lacking amongst some healthcare workers, reinforcing and contributing to pre-existing barriers to healthcare access.[4,21]

The challenge in primary care is to appreciate the unique health profile of the Traveller community. In this way health services can be modified, through local needs assessment, and so can actually deliver care in an appropriate and culturally sensitive manner.[1]

Health problems

There are not enough studies that focus on the health of Gypsies and Travellers in the UK. Some studies have found that Traveller communities 'self-report' a significantly higher number of medical problems, including a higher prevalence of respiratory problems (asthma, bronchitis), chest pain, arthritis, and anxiety and depression.[3]

Goward *et al.* suggest that a more joined-up approach to mental health services for Gypsies and Travellers is required, with improvements in communication across social and economic boundaries.[21] Various stressors may contribute to the high levels of 'self-reported' anxiety and depression (three and two times more than the general population respectively), with women more likely to experience these mental health problems.[3] These stressors may include changes to Travelling patterns, placement in fixed, residential housing,[14] uncertainties regarding eviction[3] and bereavements within the close-knit Traveller network.[2]

Women's health and maternal care is a concern considering the high 'self-reported' rates of miscarriage and poor health access during pregnancy.[10] The Confidential Enquiry into Maternal and Child Health (CEMACH) reported that the rates of maternal death in the UK were greatest amongst Traveller communities, and in most cases could have been preventable.[22]

Childhood immunisation uptake is known to be low.[10] While barriers to health are discussed later in this chapter, some contributory factors include personal and cultural views about the value and need of immunisation and difficulties with follow-up and recall due to mobile communities.[23] Considering the GP curriculum (statement 2.04), it is important to have an understanding of the local community and tailor services appropriately such as outreach programmes, opportunistic treatment and appropriate health material that the target group can understand.[23] Bearing all this in mind, a parent still has a right to refuse[23] but appropriate steps should be taken to be sure that his or her decision is informed. In addition, a small study in the UK demonstrated that amongst Travelling communities there was a low prevalence of dental registration uptake. Registration was largely influenced by the mobile nature of some Travelling communities, who were less likely to access preventive dental services.[24]

Overall, these initial studies demonstrate that health problems do exist in this patient group that require prevention, intervention and management tailored to their unique needs. In the course of Travelling, brief encounters with healthcare services may only permit time for acute management as opposed to proactive care such as childhood surveillance, screening[12] and routine dental care.[24]

Case scenario 1 is fictional and will illustrate the differences in patient and clinician agenda and concerns. The role of specialised health advocates may also bridge communication between this unique patient group and primary care healthcare workers.

....

Case scenario 1

Niamh is a 62-year-old Irish Traveller. She had been an active Traveller, up until her husband died three years ago.

Although supported by her daughters, she was unable to keep up the Traveller lifestyle on her own. Fortunately, she lives on an authorised site and is happy to remain in the caravan she shared with her husband.

Since the death of her husband she says her 'nerves' have been troubling her and tells the health visitor about this.

During a review with the doctor, she seems objectively low. She also coughs intermittently and seems a little dyspnoeic.

Niamh dismisses her chronic cough, saying it's only a small problem that doesn't affect her activities for the day. She attributes this to her many Travelling years.

Niamh agrees to counselling sessions at the practice to discuss her 'nerves' further but is not keen on any medication. She permits examination of her chest – there are a few basal crepitations – but declines any further investigations as it is too much fuss and she can still manage her daily chores. If she has any problems she will raise them with the health visitor next time.

....

Learning points

▷ The close Traveller community can mean that bereavement is felt much more acutely. Likewise, the proximity to extended family and friends can be protective and supportive. Mental health problems such as anxiety and depression may be more prevalent, underreported or simply unaddressed.

▷ The use of health visitors/advocates who are culturally aware of Gypsy/Traveller customs is desirable. GPs may identify 'cultural awareness' as a personal development need.

▷ It is important to remember that the patient's agenda and concerns may be different from those of the GP. In this case, it would be important to address the patient's 'nerves' but also exclude important red flags concerning her chronic cough, try (or plan) to address her health concerns as well as respecting her decision to defer further investigations. Offering reassurance about possible treatment options dependent on the working diagnosis may be helpful.

....

Health beliefs: impact of culture and perceptions

Health beliefs influence how Travellers view and make decisions about their health. It is the physician's responsibility to identify and understand how a patient's health belief may impact on the care the GP gives. Some of these health beliefs are discussed below.

The Travelling Way

The ability to travel is largely perceived, by Travellers, as beneficial to health,[25,26] where those who rarely travel are considered to have the poorest health.[3] Traveller communities usually live on sites, in close proximity to family, extended family and friends. Due to a shortage of authorised settlements, the option to continue this nomadic tradition is under particular threat[4] and the threat of eviction may itself contribute to anxieties.

Moving into conventional housing is also often associated with a poorer health state, chronic illness and anxiety in Traveller communities.[3] Conversely, some make the choice to settle in houses if they believe that the Traveller lifestyle has contributed to their ill health.[3,26] Although certain benefits of conventional housing are recognised, such as stability, security and ready access to basic amenities,[12] the trade-off is a sense of social isolation[25] and the culture shock that comes with not living the Traveller lifestyle any more.[26] This may also feed into feelings of stress, anxiety and panic,[26] as described by one interviewed Gypsy: 'and when you're closed in and you're shut in behind … 'cos where I'm so used to travelling … and you just shut that door behind you and you just think to yourself, that's it, I'm locked in'.[26]

Fatalism is 'the belief that all events in life are predetermined and inevitable'.[26] This view is a common attitude to illness in Traveller groups, where medical problems are considered as one's fate and destined to happen, regardless of the intervention of a physician.[3] This fatalistic view can also influence areas such as 'health promotion and education', which rely largely on not only the provision of care but also engagement of the targeted group.[26] As such, Traveller groups may have a reduced incentive to partake in screening and immunisation programmes if they see this supposed 'preventive' step as futile.[11,26]

Fatalist views can be further perpetuated by fears around particular diagnosis, e.g. cancer and the fear of death.[3,5] Such fears are often passed down verbally through the generations, in a similar fashion to information regarding their history, unchanged and unchallenged.[25] As a result, beliefs and behaviours about medical problems may be maintained.[3,23,26]

The presence of these factors can lead to avoidance of 'the problem' and its management,[3] and ultimately late presentation and diagnosis if the patient is to change his or her mind. Unfortunately, this may further reinforce fatality if presentation is so late as to offer a poor prognosis.[26]

In a similar vein, religion plays an influential part in the lives of Travellers. For example, Irish Travellers are commonly associated with Catholicism. With regards to 'fatalism', Travellers may believe that their fate has already been predetermined by God but also that they may turn to God or seek spiritual support for help through difficult times, such as illness.[3]

Low expectations of health and tolerance

Despite having numerous or significant symptoms, Travellers may well 'normalise and accept' their ill health,[25] especially if they are still able to function and perform their normal activities.[3,25] Because of poor access to health care generally, Travellers may also not appreciate the significance of certain symptoms,[25] although this problem is not unique to this group and could be managed with appropriate health promotion.

....

Case scenario 2

Kate is 22 years' old, married and pregnant with her second child. Ethnically she is a Romany Gypsy.

She is a full-time mum and has just recently moved into a one-bedroom flat with her husband and 3-year-old daughter. She is happy to be settled in a home, after facing eviction from the site, although she misses the fact that her family and extended family are not close to her now.

She registers at the local general practice and needs some help filling in the paperwork because she struggles a little to read.

This pregnancy is unplanned. They have always used the withdrawal method; her husband has never been keen on other types of contraception. Kate thinks that she is 16 weeks' pregnant now.

She previously lived on an unauthorised site, near the local sewage works, and has only been able to register as a temporary resident with previous GPs. She wasn't aware that she could access free routine dental care while pregnant, but in any case she had never been registered with a dentist.

She is unaware of her own or her daughter's immunisation history but there was a strong feeling amongst the other mothers in the community that immunisation was not needed and that some immunisations were harmful. She felt her last pregnancy was okay and reports no problems.

Kate wonders if the close proximity to a sewage works will affect this pregnancy.

The doctor takes her booking bloods and refers her for further antenatal care. Kate agrees to be seen by a health visitor at home who will discuss some of the concerns she has regarding immunisations. Her daughter's development seems appropriate and the doctor can only reassure Kate at this stage.

....

Learning outcomes

▷ Gypsies and Travellers may feel isolated if moving away from their normal Travelling environments. It is important to consider the possible mental health problems such as anxiety and low mood.

▷ Temporary residents do not have reliable or maintained medical records. This can make decisions about care difficult if historical information is not available.

▷ Gypsies and Travellers may not be aware of free additional services or what they provide, such as dental care and health visiting.

▷ It is important that further information regarding Kate's antenatal care is given in a format she can understand. Some Gypsies and Travellers have low literacy levels and it may be helpful to signpost to local educational services to help address this.

▷ Again, here it is important to understand the underlying cultural beliefs that influence health behaviour.

....

Other issues include gender preferences, and the culture of Travellers not to talk about very personal issues, e.g. women's health.[22,25]

Case scenario 2 is a fictional case exploring the difficulties from a mobile community, where contact with primary care services may not be traditional. Health education has to be considered in a way that this patient group can access and understand, and being aware of common cultural beliefs can help facilitate a tailored and more helpful consultation.

Access and provision: barriers to health care

There is a range of barriers that prevent access to health care. We know that it 'is common for socially excluded groups to have low health aspirations, poor expectations of services and limited opportunities to shape their care'[11] and, as such, even with the right infrastructure patients may not present. The expectation of discrimination will remain a constant problem until the trust of Traveller communities is gained through continual efforts to include them.[12] Further, all staff should have ongoing training that includes cultural competency.

Findings from Irish Traveller studies demonstrate a lower life expectancy in Traveller groups, with women living 12 years' less, and men 10 years' less than the same groups in the general population.[9] Similar data are unfortunately not available in Britain, although some studies demonstrate that, if Traveller communities have good access to public services, life expectancy is comparable to the surrounding, general population.[12]

Being a Traveller poses a practical barrier[3] and, by default, not having permanent accommodation is an initial problem because many GPs will not register patients without a permanent address. However, it should be noted that access to primary NHS health care in the UK is based on residency and not on a permanent postal address.[1] In addition, Gypsies and Travellers still face the same problems with access to health care regardless of their accommodation type.[4] Like other vulnerable groups, Travellers have the right to be fully registered with an NHS general practice unless the list is full or the person resides outside the practice boundary. Note that it is not acceptable to refuse 'persons applying for registration for reasons relating to the applicant's race, gender, social class, age, religion, sexual orientation, appearance, disability or medical condition'.[27]

Consideration has to be given to the poor literacy levels in Traveller groups.[12] Already disadvantaged by unaddressed cultural views, health promotion and provision should be delivered in a format that Traveller communities can understand.[24] Communication difficulties between health workers and Travellers have been observed and this further fuels a need for increased cultural awareness.[3] The role of the specialised health visitor (as well as other healthcare workers) in respecting and understanding the Traveller culture, being a constant and regular feature, and also an advocate for Travellers has been beneficial in managing suspicion and distrust of non-Travellers.[3] This quote taken from Van Cleemput and Parry illustrates this: 'it was important that someone who had already gained [the Gypsy's] trust facilitated the introduction. ... The Health Visitor taught the researcher about the history so that he not inadvertently offend anyone through ignorance of their beliefs and way of life.'[4]

For Travellers who are actually aware of, and identify deficiencies in, health care, some responsibility will lie with them to raise the issues of concern. However, therein lies the problem of engagement and trust, and the underlying cultural and health beliefs that influence effective dialogue between Travellers and healthcare workers. Tackling barriers to health care is multifactorial and rarely can one problem be managed on its own. It is important for the health professional to recognise these barriers in order to understand the patient's reluctance to what may be seen as 'conventional' treatment and management options.

Conclusions: addressing inequality

Choosing Health, a Department of Health white paper, described three guiding principles in empowering patients to make healthy choices:

1. Informed choice

2. Personalisation

3. Partnership working between service providers and users.[28]

Improving health outcomes in Traveller communities remains complex because Traveller health models are very different from the traditional medical models that are already in place. Wider research and local needs assessments will facilitate a greater understanding of their unique health needs, and, more importantly, how best to manage them.

The PCSF[1] and the Department of Health's *Inclusion Health* document[11] are a useful armoury in planning the commissioning of services for Gypsies and Travellers.

Some key points, from these documents, are mentioned here:

- **building trust and understanding with Traveller communities** – a sensitivity to the origin of Traveller cultures, beliefs and history is needed as well as active management of discrimination

- **cultural awareness** – training in this area should be considered as it remains fundamental to understanding the presentation and management of illness and disease. Healthcare workers should be aware of resources to improve awareness [10,25]

- **permitting access to mainstream primary care services** – issues with regards to registration should be clarified and access for minority or marginalised groups should be promoted

- **Equality Impact Assessments (EqIAs)** – there should be an assessment of local needs so that services can be modified or streamlined to facilitate access

- **involvement of Gypsy and Traveller communities** – at all stages, Traveller communities should be involved in their own care.

Public organisations have a responsibility to ethnic minority groups to promote equality and develop strategies to combat inequalities.[1,5] A need to respect and reflect values is essential in gaining the trust of these patient groups, and effecting positive changes.

Useful resources

- Equality and Human Rights Commission, www.equalityhumanrights.com. Has the statutory responsibility to protect, promote and enforce equality across several key areas.

- Gypsy Roma Traveller Leeds, www.gypsyromatravellerleeds.co.uk/.

- Race Equality Foundation, www.raceequalityfoundation.org.uk. Independent charity concerned with interventions that would overcome discrimination in health, housing and social care.

References

1. Primary Care Service Framework: Gypsy & Traveller communities, 19 May 2009, www.pcc-cic. org.uk/sites/default/files/articles/attachments/ehrg_gypsies_and_travellers_pcsf_190509.pdf [accessed July 2013].

2. Matthews Z. *The Health of Gypsies and Travellers in the UK* (Better Health Briefing 12). London: Race Equality Foundation, 2008.

3. Parry G, Van Cleemput P, Peters J, *et al*. *Health Status of Gypsies & Travellers in England: report of Department of Health Inequalities in Health Research Initiative Project 121/75000*. Sheffield: University of Sheffield, 2004.

4. Van Cleemput P, Parry G. Health status of Gypsy Travellers. *Journal of Public Health* 2001; **23 (2)**: 129–34.

5. HM Government. Race Relations Act 1976. www.legislation.gov.uk/ukpga/1976/74/pdfs/ ukpga_19760074_en.pdf   [accessed July 2013].

6. Commission for Racial Equality. *Common Ground: equality, good race relations and sites for Gypsies and Irish Travellers*. London: CRE, 2006.

7. Office for National Statistics. 2011 Census, key statistics for local authorities in England and Wales. www.ons.gov.uk/ons/publications/re-reference-tables.html?edition=tcm%3A77-286262 [accessed October 2013].

8. Hajioff S, McKee M. The health of the Roma people: a review of the published literature. *Journal of Epidemiology and Community Health* 2000; **54**: 864–9.

9. Department of Health and Children. *Traveller Health: a national strategy 2002–2005*. Dublin: Department of Health, 2002.

10. Parry G, Van Cleemput P, Peters J, *et al*. Health status of Gypsies & Travellers in England. *Journal of Epidemiology and Community Health* 2007; **61**: 198–204.

11. Department of Health. *Inclusion Health: improving primary care for socially excluded people*. London: DH, 2010.

12. Cemlyn S, Greenfields M, Burnett S, *et al*. *Inequalities Experienced by Gypsy and Traveller Communities: a review*. London: Equality and Human Rights Commission, 2009.

13. Barton H, Grant M. A health map for the local human habitat. *Journal for the Royal Society for the Promotion of Health* 2006; **126 (6)**: 252–3.

14. Lane P, Tribe R. Towards an understanding of the cultural health needs of older gypsies: an introduction. *Working with Older People* 2010; **14(2)**: 23–30.

15. Home Office. Criminal Justice and Public Order Act 1994. Circular 4511994. London: Home Office, 1994.

16. HM Government. Race Relations (Amendment) Act 2000. www.legislation.gov.uk/ukpga/2000/34/pdfs/ukpga_20000034_en.pdf   [accessed July 2013].

17. Decade of Roma Inclusion, www.romadecade.org.

18. Royal College of General Practitioners. *The GP Consultation in Practice* (Curriculum Statement 2.01). London: RCGP, 2012.

19. Royal College of General Practitioners. *Enhancing Professional Knowledge* (Curriculum Statement 2.04). London: RCGP, 2012.

20. Royal College of General Practitioners. *Healthy People: promoting health and preventing disease* (Curriculum Statement 3.01). London: RCGP, 2012.

21. Goward P, Repper J, Appleton L, *et al.* Crossing boundaries: identifying and meeting the mental health needs of Gypsies and Travellers. *Journal of Mental Health* 2006; **15(3)**: 315–27.

22. Department of Health. *Why Mothers Die: report on the confidential enquiries into maternal deaths in the United Kingdom 1994–1996*. London: TSO, 2001.

23. Feder G, Vaclavik T, Streetly A. Traveller Gypsies and childhood immunization: a study in east London. *British Journal of General Practice* 1993; **43(372)**: 281–4.

24. Edwards DM, Watt RG. Oral health care in the lives of Gypsy Travellers in east Hertfordshire. *British Dental Journal* 1997; **183(7)**: 252–7.

25. Van Cleemput P, Parry G, Thomas K, *et al.* Health-related beliefs and experiences of Gypsies and Travellers: a qualitative study. *Journal of Epidemiology and Community Health* 2007; **61(3)**: 205–10.

26. Dion X. Gypsies and Travellers: cultural influences on health. *Community Practitioner* 2008; **81(6)**: 31–4.

27. Asylum seekers and vulnerable migrants. RCGP Position Statement. January 2013. www.rcgp.org.uk/policy/rcgp-policy-areas/asylum-seekers-and-vulnerable-migrants.aspx [accessed July 2013].

28. HM Government. *Choosing Health: making healthy choices easier. Executive summary*. London: DH, 2004.

5

Refugees and asylum seekers in primary care
From looking after to working together

Gervase Vernon and Rayah Feldman

Aim

Many GPs and other members of the primary care team will be looking after refugees and asylum seekers in their practices. Some refugees will have arrived recently; others arrived long ago and are settled in this country. This chapter outlines resources available to refugees in primary care and reviews the evidence of their effectiveness where it is available. It will discuss the role of specialist services and those available within mainstream general practice.[1]

Key learning points

- Define asylum and refugee status, and the process of seeking this status.

- Describe the health status of refugees and asylum seekers.

- Be aware of services available within mainstream general practice and those offered by specialist services.

The GP curriculum and refugees

Care of refugees and asylum seekers is not mentioned specifically in the RCGP curriculum. Equally, most curriculum statements have some relevance to the care of this group. The interpretive statement with the most direct relevance is statement 2.01 *The GP Consultation in Practice.*[2]

Introduction

Primary care for refugees is, in important ways, like primary care for all patients. There are only likely to be ten minutes available for the consultation. Patients' expectations may be unrealistic; their needs are many and various, and not all are medical. Some of the services to which the practitioner might wish to refer the patient are underfunded or absent. Yet a kind smile and time spent listening will be accepted with gratitude.

It is at the core of general practice to elicit the health beliefs and expectations of the patient and, in this respect, consultations with refugees are no different. Indeed, in some ways this can be easier with refugees.

This is because we expect that their beliefs will be different from our own and therefore the need to explore health beliefs is clear. With UK-born patients it is often easier to assume that they share our own beliefs so that we fail to check that the patients share them, and end up giving advice that is based on beliefs that the patients do not share or perhaps even do not understand. Equally, expectations of health care will be different and this applies especially to the divide between primary and secondary care.[3]

The evidence base for their care is mainly from descriptive studies. Further details are available at http://repository.forcedmigration.org/pdf/?pid=fmo:5934, which is an archived version of this chapter with more extensive references.[4]

Current situation

Since 1945 war, civil unrest, human rights violations and natural disasters have led to large numbers of people seeking refuge in other countries, or being internally displaced in their own countries. The United Nations High Commissioner for Refugees estimated that there were 11.4 million refugees and asylum seekers worldwide in 2007.[5] Two-thirds of the world's refugees live in developing countries, with only 21% in Europe, and less than 3% or about 270,000 in the UK.[6] In 2011 the top four countries of origin of asylum seekers in the UK were Iran, Pakistan, Sri Lanka and Afghanistan.[7,8] The number of applications for asylum in Britain have fallen dramatically in recent years from 84,000 in 2002 to 18,000 in 2010.[9] In general 20–30% of asylum seekers have been awarded refugee status or leave to stay on humanitarian grounds.

Refugees are only a small proportion of the migrants living in Britain (see Table 5.1). There are about 2.8 million legal migrants[10] and an estimated half a million irregular migrant workers,[10] many in the hotel and hospitality industry in the southeast. There has recently been large-scale legal migration from the EU, especially Eastern Europe. Other irregular migrants include dependants and visa overstayers. There are also an unknown number of failed asylum seekers who have not been removed or cannot be removed from the UK. Where migration is illegal, almost by definition numbers can only be guesses, but they give an idea of the scale of the problem to those unfamiliar with this area.

Table 5.1 **Approximate numbers of various categories of migrants in the UK**

	Legal status	Numbers (best guess)	Employment rights	Other rights
Economic migrants (legal)	Legal	2.8 million	Yes	Some
Migrants with 'irregular' papers	Irregular	500,000	No	Few
Asylum seekers	Legal (under international treaty, the Geneva Convention)	20,000	No	Substantial
Refugees	Legal		Yes	As UK citizens
'Failed asylum seekers'	Variable	Greater than 100,000	No	Few

Source: numbers based on references in the text above.

Definitions

The 1951 UN Refugee Convention (Geneva Convention), to which the UK government is a signatory, defines a *refugee* as someone outside his or her own country and unable to return as a result of a well-founded fear of persecution on grounds of race, religion, nationality, political opinion or membership of a social group.[11] Until April 2006 a person accepted as a refugee under the Geneva Convention was granted refugee status and Indefinite Leave to Remain (ILR) in the UK. Since then a refugee is given temporary status for five years with permanent status only granted if he or she is still considered to be at risk at the end of this period.[11]

In the UK an *asylum seeker* is a person seeking recognition as a refugee who has submitted an application for protection under the Geneva Convention and is waiting for the claim to be decided by the Home Office. This includes people who have made an initial application, or who have had an initial application refused and are awaiting an appeal or a decision from an appeal. They may have asylum seeker status for several years as there are many stages to the appeal process, and during the last decade many asylum decisions have taken a very long time to resolve.

Most asylum seekers are not granted refugee status but before April 2003 could be granted Exceptional Leave to Remain (ELR) for up to four years. Since April 2003 ELR was replaced by Humanitarian Protection (HP) and Discretionary Leave (DL). HP grants leave for five years to people who face breaches of human rights under Article 3 of the European Convention on Human Rights (ECHR) relating to inhuman or degrading treatment or punishment. DL grants leave for three years under Article 8 of the

ECHR, which covers the right to private and family life. Unaccompanied minors are granted DL until they reach age 18. After these periods their status must be reviewed and they are expected to return to their country if the situation there improves. This situation can give rise to further protracted appeals.

A *failed asylum seeker* is a person whose asylum application has been refused and who is deemed to have exhausted all available channels for appeal. However, many such people are pursuing further legal challenges as Home Office decisions may be wrong, for instance where the Home Office has failed to take account of its own Gender Guidance[12] or where circumstances have been identified that were not taken into account in the initial decision or appeal. Some are simply unable to go back to their home country.[13,14]

The triple trauma of the refugee

Refugees go through many difficulties. These have been categorised into phases (Table 5.2) by Prof. Baker from the refugee studies programme at the University of Oxford – the 'triple trauma of the refugee'.[15] The first phase is the trauma in the country of origin, a trauma so severe that the refugee decides to leave his or her home. The second trauma is the trauma endured during migration where refugees may travel arduously overland or by air with false or no documentation in fear of what will happen to them on arrival. The third trauma is the trauma of resettlement in the host country.

Table 5.2 **Baker's triple trauma of the refugee**

Trauma	Responsibility of host country authorities?
In country of origin	No
During flight and migration	No
In host country	Yes

Source: Baker R. Psychosocial consequences for tortured refugees seeking asylum and refugee status in Europe.[15]

There have been attempts to quantify the relative importance of these factors.[16] Recent studies have shown that the health of refugees can worsen after reaching the UK,[17-19] particularly their mental health. One of us has described the 'Home Office syndrome' brought on by long periods of uncertainty waiting to find out one's eventual status.[20] We have also reviewed the policy options followed in other countries and in the central administration of the EU.[21]

The asylum process in the UK

It is worth describing in more detail what happens to asylum seekers after arrival in the UK, because the stage they have reached in this process will affect their interaction with primary care. It should be borne in mind that successfully completing the difficult journey to the UK proves qualities of resourcefulness and resilience that bode well for eventual integration into and contribution to the host society.

In 2005 the government introduced a 'New Asylum Model' (NAM) to deal with asylum applications.[22] Under the NAM applicants have a screening interview as soon as they lodge their asylum claim. They are then allocated to one of a range of tracks through which their claim is processed. The most important difference between tracks is between applicants who are 'fast-tracked' and those who are given temporary admission into the UK. Fast-tracked applicants, largely determined by nationality, are detained in immigration centres while their claim is processed within tight deadlines. Applicants who are not detained have to complete a Statement of Evidence Form within ten working days, giving their reasons for claiming asylum. This form is then used as the basis for a full asylum interview. This interview is taken as the basis of the claim for asylum. Any subsequent changes are seen as evidence of unreliability.

Yet the first interview with a government official may well not reflect the full story. A refugee may have fled his or her home because of physical, including sexual, violence and torture from government agents or others and may still be traumatised from the experiences he or she has suffered. The Home Office's own Gender Guidance requires sensitive treatment of women who may have experienced sexual violence, but a recent study shows that this guidance is often not followed.[12,23] Brain injury, malnutrition, depression and post-traumatic stress disorder (PTSD) may impair accurate recall.[24] Moreover, the culture at the Home Office has been described as a 'culture of disbelief'.[25]

Following the interview the asylum seekers may be dealt with under the Fast Track procedure and detained under a tight timetable with very limited time for appeal against refusal.[26] Those not detained in this way are entitled to support by the UKBA (the Home Office UK Border Agency). Support rates are based on 70% of the Income Support levels, so, for example, a single adult in receipt of cash support currently receives £36.62 per week.[27] The UKBA also provides accommodation for asylum seekers in dispersal areas outside London and the southeast. Refugees who are receiving treatment from Freedom from Torture (formerly the Medical Foundation for the Care of Victims of Torture) or a few other types of treatment can apply not to be dispersed from London.

There may follow months or years of appeals. Asylum seekers currently have no right to work though they may apply after 12 months to have the conditions of their stay changed to enable them to seek employment.

During the asylum process a proportion of asylum seekers are detained, some in detention centres and some in prisons, although they have been charged with no crime. This proportion has been estimated at 10% and may be higher in asylum seekers of particular nationalities.[28] Britain is the only European country where asylum seekers can be detained indefinitely and without judicial review.[28] Detention can be judicially reviewed if lawyers believe the detention is illegal or bail has been refused for unjustified reasons. There is no automatic judicial review.

What primary care is available?

Entitlement to primary care

Asylum seekers are entitled to NHS treatment without charge for as long as their applications (including appeals) are under consideration and they can thus apply to register with a GP.[29,30] They can also apply for free prescriptions in England using form HC2. This form will be given to asylum seekers by the UKBA when they receive asylum support. Both asylum seekers and anyone given leave to remain are exempt from charges for NHS hospital treatment.

Currently GP practices have the discretion to accept failed asylum seekers as registered NHS patients. This is however a situation that can change and the government is currently planning changes in charging that will affect primary care.[29,30] However, uncertainty about entitlement has resulted in confusion among both asylum seekers and GPs about their rights to treatment.[31]

Secondary care is chargeable from the date the asylum claim is deemed to have failed but treatment already underway at the time when the asylum seeker's claim, including any appeals, is finally rejected should remain free of charge until completion.[29,30] Maternity care, and any immediately necessary treatment, while chargeable, must not be denied due to lack of funds. Testing for HIV and treatment of TB remain free. In an important recent change, treatment of HIV has become free.[32,33]

Peter Hall, the chair of Physicians for Human Rights UK, in a BMJ editorial, deplored the lack of access of failed asylum seekers to secondary care and pointed to its damaging consequences.[34] He questioned whether the government, and any doctor denying access to health care, was in breach of the UN International Covenant on Economic, Social and Cultural Rights (Geneva, UN, 1976). The government and any individual complying may also be in breach of EU directives.[35]

There is currently no requirement for practices to ask to see official documentation (e.g. a passport) but the Department of Health and the Refugee Council suggest that some supporting evidence of address may assist registration.[36] The situation with regard to access to health care for vulnerable migrants has recently been reviewed from a European perspective.[21,37]

Gateway services

Some services facilitate access to full registration in mainstream practices and may also provide specialist support to mainstream practitioners. They also provide information about other health services such as dentists, pharmacists and hospitals. They are not necessarily general practices and do not themselves offer comprehensive primary care services. In a review of primary care services for refugees and asylum seekers, Feldman categorised these kinds of services as 'Gateway' services.[38]

Access for refugees and asylum seekers requires health professionals to identify people who are not registered and provide them with information and often assistance about what to do. Personal Medical Services (PMS) pilots have played a major role in facilitating access to health care for this group both in dispersal areas and in other places by means of dedicated practices or specialist refugee clinics in general practice.[38,39] Such practices, specialist health teams or nurse-led outreach services provide one gateway to primary care registration. These services can provide treatment to refugees and asylum seekers in hostels and health centres, and liaise with GPs to get patients registered in mainstream services. Some use hand-held records to facilitate continuity of care.[40]

Where no dedicated services are yet in place, specialist staff can play a crucial coordinating role in ensuring access to services, monitoring need, and providing support to front-line health workers responsible for delivering care. This may involve support for asylum seekers and GPs, and developing information systems to check that people are registered. Some Primary Care Trusts/Organisations (formerly called PCTs but now replaced by Clinical Commissioning Groups [CCGs]) in England employ specialist health visitors for asylum seekers. They work across an area as well as with dedicated practices to facilitate GP and dentist registration for refugees and asylum seekers.[41]

Core services

By 'core' services we mean general practice. Core services are normally provided in mainstream practices with no specialist provision but can be provided in dedicated practices.

Most dedicated practices are funded as PMS with a local contract with a CCG to provide a dedicated service, or simply to give special services to refugees. Special services to refugees can now be funded under the new GMS contract (nGMS) via a 'local enhanced service' in a mainstream practice. These arrangements will continue to change as the health service evolves.

Dedicated practices for asylum seekers, many of which are nurse-led, serve a local population of asylum seekers or particular accommodation centers or hostels. They often also serve other vulnerable population groups, especially homeless people. They offer a wide range of services to their patients, beginning with full registration and comprehensive health assessments. Other services such as TB screening and vaccination depend on the staffing levels and facilities available. Dedicated practices usually have a holistic approach to health care, providing multidisciplinary services and offering more time to patients.[36]

In dispersal areas, such practices maintain strong links with housing providers, who are their main initial contact with patients. Most have well-established links with social care services and with others such as child care or baby clinics to which patients are referred when appropriate.[42,43]

While dedicated practices offer useful solutions where there are large numbers of refugees and asylum seekers, they also risk becoming redundant if asylum seekers are dispersed elsewhere or if the numbers coming into the area they serve are reduced. Thus health commissioners face a choice between funding specialised services or existing mainstream services.

Support services

There are two main types of support services: those concerned with facilitating communication and information, including health promotion, and those providing specialist care, especially in mental health and for survivors of trauma. All require training and support for health professionals.

Support services facilitating communication and information

Refugee health teams and dedicated practices, particularly, see involvement with local communities as part of their remit and as essential to facilitate access for members of refugee communities. Community-based organisations can contribute significantly to planning more appropriate and acceptable services, and can be the source of interpreters, advocates and link workers.[44] Language is a major barrier both to accessing primary care and to reporting health problems.[45,46] A common solution is for relatives to interpret on the patient's behalf. This has serious limitations, especially regarding confidentiality and sexual health, let alone allegations of rape or torture. Professional interpreters are to be preferred for these cases, though issues of gender and ethnic or political grouping will still arise (see Table 5.3).

Table 5.3 **Use of interpreters**

	Cost	Suitable for minor illness	Suitable for gynaecological problems/rape or torture
Family interpreters	Free	Yes	No
Telephone interpreting	High	Yes	No
Professional interpreters	High	Yes	Yes, with limitations

A good interpreter is also an advocate: explaining the patient's world to the doctor and the doctor's world to the patient. Two sites for translated materials are listed in the resource list at the end of the chapter.

Resources with translated materials exist, but they change rapidly.

Support services for mental health and services for survivors of torture and organised violence

There is widespread agreement that there is a shortage of appropriate mental health services to meet the needs of refugees and asylum seekers.[47,48]

There are a limited number of specialist services for refugees and asylum seekers run by Mental Health Trusts or by independent bodies.[36] Some trauma services include survivors of torture or violent conflicts within their remit. Freedom from Torture offers both physical and mental health services for this group (www.freedomfromtorture.org.) However, such services may not be available to refugees and asylum seekers with more general mental health problems. Where there is very high demand for existing services, or where no specialist services exist, partnerships have been or are being developed between a number of agencies to provide services for this group.[49]

Health needs and the provision of services within general practice

Most mental health care for refugees is provided within general practice and good-practice guides exist.[50,51] The Royal College of Psychiatrists has recently reviewed the mental health care of asylum seekers and refugees.[52] A small minority of refugees and asylum seekers suffer from well-defined mental illnesses such as schizophrenia for which there is standard treatment but most just feel great distress and anxiety, which may not require medical treatment. One study suggests that a lack of social support is a stronger predictor of distress than trauma factors.[53]

Many reports advocate social and practical support to address refugees' mental health problems and several partnership initiatives have been developed with refugee community groups to support social as well as counselling services with their members.[54] This can also help to avoid the stigmatisation of mental illness that exists in many cultures.

Some professionals attribute much distress among refugees and asylum seekers to PTSD as a specific illness. Guidance is available.[55]

Physical illness is also common in refugees. It must be distinguished from mental distress, which is often expressed in physical symptoms such as headache or whole-body pain. Cultural expectations of early referral for hospital tests or treatment are likely to be more of a challenge than difficulty in diagnosis (see Table 5.4 for some examples).

Table 5.4 **Common stress-related symptoms in asylum seekers and refugees**

Symptoms	Exclude serious disease
Gastritis	Duodenal ulcer
Headaches	Epilepsy non-disclosed
Backache	Disc prolapse
Whole-body pain	Arthritis, vitamin D deficiency
Frequent infections	HIV
Shortness of breath	Asthma
Palpitations	Rheumatic heart disease
Dermatitis	Scabies, tropical infections
Vulvovaginitis	STDs, non-disclosed rape

Note: with thanks to Dr Lawson, personal communication.

Antenatal care for refugee women poses specific problems and a useful training pack is available from Medact (a charity involved in policies that affect global health issues). Women refugees suffer from a range of gender-specific problems, including after-effects of rape, and HIV as it affects women.[56] Feldman has written a guide to commissioning services to these women.[57–59] Female genital mutilation (FGM) is common in a belt of sub-Saharan Africa running from Somalia to West Africa.[60] Many of the women in the UK with FGM are from Somalia. Clearly a good interpreter and cultural sensitivity are required in raising these issues with women. The wishes of individual women will vary.[61] The treatment, if desired, is surgical, and the key issue is to operate before the woman goes into labour. Hence a reversal operation (deinfibulation) before pregnancy is highly desirable; if pregnant, the operation should be planned at 20 weeks rather than undertaken as an emergency during labour.[61]

When consulting with a refugee or asylum seeker, the GP must also bear in mind other medical conditions that can arise from the country of origin of the patient (i.e. tropical disease) or are unmasked in their host country (i.e. vitamin D deficiency).

Different perspectives

To understand the politics of primary health care for refugees and asylum seekers it is worth recognising the different perspectives and expectations of stakeholders. Most GPs have a humanitarian outlook and are willing to look after refugees but, according to a BMA survey, they would wish to be paid, to have the time and the training to do the job, and to have services to which they may refer.[62] Refugees' expectations of health care may reflect unfamiliarity with GP services, especially the need for booking and appointments in primary care rather than immediate hospital treatment. Mental illness and epilepsy may be more strongly stigmatised than in the host community. Existing patients' ability to access GPs must also be considered.

There is anecdotal evidence that providing dedicated services for asylum seekers risks generating resentment among the original patients in a practice or locality. The government's health policy is to provide a broad spectrum of services but in practice provision reflects concerns both with cost of provision and with public health. It may also be influenced by the government's desire not to appear 'soft' on asylum seekers.[63]

Understanding how it feels to be a refugee

Treating refugees in primary care requires not only the information of the sort provided in this chapter and the use of interpreters, but also the ability to understand how a refugee views the world. We believe this can be taught and in a number of ways. If the practice is one with many refugees then the doctor can learn directly from them. Clearly, stories of refugees in literature or films will be helpful for some.[64] For others the refugee's point of view can be understood via a tutorial. Here, the trick is to encourage the registrar to find a suitable memory, such as one of migration or a first day at boarding school. The doctor's own feelings from that time will suggest the feelings that refugees are likely to be experiencing now. With luck, the doctor will experience a moment of illumination and empathy.[65]

Conclusion

We have tried to describe the current situation of refugees in the UK and their journey through the healthcare system. There is a tension between the provision of specialised services, most appropriate at the beginning of the asylum process, and the provision of services in main-stream primary care, which may facilitate integration and allow more continuity of care. Finally we have highlighted a number of resources that may be helpful to all primary care teams caring for these migrants.

Applied Knowledge Test (AKT) questions

Which of the following statements is/are true?

1 The asylum journey

a The UKBA sets the support it gives to asylum seekers at 70% or less of what a similar UK citizen would get.

b Asylum seekers (who receive full UKBA support) may choose where to live in the UK.

c Asylum seekers are entitled to work.

d Under UK asylum procedures both children and adults may be detained indefinitely and without judicial review.

2 TB

a It is government policy to screen asylum seekers for TB.

b TB treatment is free even to failed asylum seekers.

c All people with TB are infectious and should be segregated from the community.

d Children of asylum seekers, who are born in the UK, should have BCG vaccination in infancy.

3 Female issues

a Antenatal care is free for failed asylum seekers.

b Vitamin D deficiency is a common and treatable cause of 'whole-body pain' in women.

c A Somali woman presents for antenatal care. Vaginal examination shows that she has fused labia (due to female circumcision, FGM). No attempt should be made to reverse the operation before the onset of labour.

d Family interpreters are suitable for gynaecological problems.

4 Access

a Asylum seekers (during their asylum process) have access to the same medical facilities as UK residents, including free treatment in primary and secondary care, and free prescriptions.

b 'Failed asylum seekers', that is asylum seekers who have exhausted the appeals process, are entitled to secondary care without charge.

c 'Failed asylum seekers' are entitled to anti-HIV treatment without charge.

d 'Failed asylum seekers' are entitled to emergency care and primary care without charge.

Answers: **1 = a, d | 2 = a, b, d | 3 = b | 4 = a, d**

Useful resources

- Vernon G, Feldman R, Wamalwa A. Refugees and asylum seekers in primary care: from looking after to working together. 2006. http://repository.forcedmigration.org/pdf/?pid=fmo:5934 [accessed July 2013] – web version of the review on which this chapter is based.

- Burnett A, Fassil Y. *Meeting the Health Needs of Refugees and Asylum Seekers in the UK: an information and resource pack for health workers.* London: DH, 2002, http://webarchive.nationalarchives.gov.uk/+/www.dh.gov.uk/en/Publicationsandstatistics/Publications/PublicationsPolicyAndGuidance/DH_4010199 [accessed July 2013].

- LanguageLine Solutions, www.languageline.co.uk – offers telephone interpreting.

- Maternity Action's 'Maternity Access and Advocacy Pack', www.maternityaction.org.uk.

- Medact, www.medact.org/ – provides a forum and there is an email list that can be joined.

- King's Fund. Reading list. Refugee health care. December 2012. www.kingsfund.org.uk/sites/files/kf/field/field_pdf/Library-reading-list-refugee-health-care-Dec2012.pdf [accessed July 2013].

- For translated materials, there is a Department of Health site, http://webarchive.nationalarchives.gov.uk/20130107105354/http://www.dh.gov.uk/en/Publicationsandstatistics/Publications/DH_4123594 [accessed July 2013], and another site with translated materials, www.healthinmylanguage.com/home.aspx [accessed July 2013].

References

1. Trafford P, Winkler F. *Refugees and Primary Care*. London: RCGP, 2000.

2. Royal College of General Practitioners. *The GP Consultation in Practice* (Curriculum Statement 2.01). London: RCGP, 2012.

3. O'Donnell C, Higgins M, Chauhan R, *et al*. Asylum seekers' expectations of and trust in general practice: a qualitative study. *British Journal of General Practice* 2008; **58(557)**: 870–6.

4. Vernon G, Feldman R. Refugees and asylum seekers in primary care: from looking after to working together. 2006. http://repository.forcedmigration.org/pdf/?pid=fmo:5934 [accessed July 2013].

5. United Nations High Commissioner for Refugees. *Statistical Yearbook 2007: trends in displacement, protection and solutions*. Geneva: UNHCR, 2008.

6. Refugee Council. *Tell It Like It Is: the truth about asylum*. London: Refugee Council, 2005.

7. Refugee Council. Asylum statistics 2012. 2012. www.refugeecouncil.org.uk/assets/0001/5778/Asylum_Statistics__Aug_2012.pdf [access July 2013].

8. Home Office. *Asylum Statistics United Kingdom 2007*. London: Home Office, 2008.

9. Information Centre about Asylum and Refugees. ICAR statistics paper 1. 2009. www.icar.org.uk/ICAR%20Statistics%20Paper%201%20-%20December%202009%20update.pdf [acessed July 2013].

10. Institute for Public Policy Research. *Migration and Health in the UK*. London: IPPR, 2005, www.ippr.org.uk/ecomm/files/migration_health_factfile.pdf [accessed July 2013].

11. United Nations High Commissioner for Refugees. *The State of the World's Refugees*. Oxford: Oxford University Press, 2000.

12. Ceneda S, Palmer S. *'Lip service' or Implementation? The Home Office Gender Guidance and women's claims in the UK*. London: Asylum Aid, 2006, www.asylumaid.org.uk/data/files/publications/38/Lip_Service_or_Implementation.pdf [accessed October 2013].

13. Vernon G, Feldman R. Government proposes to end free health care for 'failed asylum seekers'. *British Journal of General Practice* 2006; **56(522)**: 59.

14. Williams P. Failed asylum seekers and access to free health care in the UK. *Lancet* 2005; **365(9473)**: 1767.

15. Baker R. Psychosocial consequences for tortured refugees seeking asylum and refugee status in Europe. In: M Basoglu (ed.). *Torture and Its Consequences: current treatment approaches*. Cambridge: Cambridge University Press, 1992, pp. 83–106.

16. Porter M, Haslam N. Predisplacement and postdisplacement factors associated with mental health of refugees and internally displaced persons: a meta-analysis. *Journal of the American Medical Association* 2005; **294(5)**: 602–12.

17. Keller A S, Rosenfeld B, Trinh-Shevrin C, *et al.* Mental health of detained asylum seekers. *Lancet* 2003; **362(9397)**: 1721–3.

18. Fazel M, Silove D. Detention of refugees. *British Medical Journal* 2006; **332(7536)**: 251–2.

19. Robjant K, Hassan R, Katona C. Mental health implications of detaining asylum seekers: systematic review. *British Journal of Psychiatry* 2009; **194(4)**: 306–12.

20. Vernon G, Ridley D, Lesetedi D. 'Home Office syndrome'. *British Journal of General Practice* 2008; **58(552)**: 510.

21. Vernon G. Denunciation: a new threat to health care for undocumented migrants. *British Journal of General Practice* 2012; **62(595)**: 98–9.

22. Refugee Forum. *The United Kingdom's Asylum System.* Ottawa: Refugee Forum, 2010.

23. Home Office. *Gender Issues in the Asylum Claim.* London: Home Office, 2006, www.ukba. homeoffice.gov.uk/sitecontent/documents/policyandlaw/asylumpolicyinstructions/apis/ gender-issue-in-the-asylum.pdf?view=Binary [accessed October 2013].

24. Cohen J. Errors of recall and credibility: can omissions and discrepancies in successive statements reasonably be said to undermine credibility of testimony? *Medicolegal Journal* 2001; **69(1)**: 25–34.

25. Webster L, Gelsthorpe L. *Deciding to Detain: how decisions to detain asylum seekers are made at ports of entry.* Cambridge: Institute of Criminology, 2000.

26. Refugee Council. *The New Asylum Model.* London: Refugee Council, 2007.

27. Office of Public Sector Information. The Asylum Support (Amendment) (No. 2) Regulations 2009. 2009.

28. Bradstock A, Trotman A. *Asylum Voices: experiences of people seeking asylum in the United Kingdom.* London: Churches Together in Britain and Ireland, 2003.

29. Department of Health. *Guidance on Implementing the Overseas Visitors Hospital Charging Regulations.* London: DH, 2011, http://webarchive.nationalarchives.gov.uk/20130513204013/ https://www.gov.uk/government/publications/implementing-the-overseas-visitors-hospital-charging-regulations-2011 [accessed October 2013].

30. Immigration Bill (HC 110), 2013, Chapter 2. www.publications.parliament.uk/pa/bills/cbill/ 2013-2014/0110/cbill_2013-20140110_en_1.htm [accessed October 2013].

31. Cohen D. New rules on treating failed asylum seekers 'do not go far enough,' says BMA. *British Medical Journal* 2009; **339**: b2982002E.

32. Department of Health. *HIV Treatment for Overseas Visitors: guidance for the NHS.* London: DH, 2012.

33. Department of Health. *Guidance on Implementing the Overseas Visitors Hospital Charging Regulations.* London: DH, 2012.

34. Hall P. Failed asylum seekers and health care. *British Medical Journal* 2006; **333(7559)**: 109–10.

35. Burnett A, Rhys-Jones D. Health care for asylum seekers. *British Medical Journal* 2006; **333**: 109–10. doi: http://dx.doi.org/10.1136/bmj.333.7559.109.

36. Department of Health, Refugee Council. *Caring for Dispersed Asylum Seekers: a resource pack.* London: DH, 2003, http://webarchive.nationalarchives.gov.uk/20130107105354/http://www.dh.gov.uk/PublicationsAndStatistics/Publications/PublicationsPolicyAndGuidance/PublicationsPolicyAndGuidanceArticle/fs/en?CONTENT_ID=4010379&chk=fsxJo5 [accessed July 2013].

37. HUMA Network. *Accesss to Health Care for Undocumented Migrants and Asylum Seekers in 10 EU Countries: law and practice.* HUMA Network, 2009.

38. Feldman R. Primary health care for refugees and asylum seekers: a review of the literature and a framework for services. *Public Health* 2006; **120(9)**: 809–16.

39. Le Feuvre P. *Adopt, Adapt and Improve: the East Kent Experience 1998–2003.* London: King's Fund, 2003.

40. Department of Health. *Personal Health Record for Asylum Applicants and Refugees.* London: DH, 2007, http://webarchive.nationalarchives.gov.uk/20130107105354/http://www.dh.gov.uk/prod_consum_dh/groups/dh_digitalassets/@dh/@en/documents/digitalasset/dh_4084549.pdf [accessed July 2013].

41. Wilson R. *Improving the Health of Asylum Seekers in Northern & Yorkshire: a report on service provision and needs.* Northern and Yorkshire Public Health Observatory, 2002.

42. North Tyneside Transitional Care Practice. *First Annual PMS Report.* Wallsend: North Tyneside Primary Care Trust, 2004.

43. Asylum Seekers and Refugee Centre for Health. *Asylum Seekers and Refugee Centre for Health Review: 06 January to 29 September 2003.* Birmingham: Asylum Seekers and Refugee Centre for Health (Birmingham), 2003.

44. Cowen T. *Suffering Alone: an examination of the mental health needs of asylum seekers and refugees in Barnet.* London: Refugee Health Access Project, Barnet Voluntary Service Council, Barnet Primary Care Trust, 2003.

45. Hunt S, Bhopal R. Self reports in research with non-English speakers. *British Medical Journal* 2003; **327(7411)**: 352–3.

46. Bischoff A, Bovier P A, Rrustemi I, *et al.* Language barriers between nurses and asylum seekers: their impact on symptom reporting and referral. *Social Science and Medicine* 2003; **57(3)**: 503–12.

47. Audit Commission. *Another Country: implementing dispersal under the Immigration and Asylum Act 1999.* London: Audit Commission for Local Authorities and the NHS in England and Wales, 2000.

48. Wilson R, Yorkshire and Humberside Refugee Support Centre. *Findings of Research into Mental Health Services for Refugees and Asylum Seekers, and Perceptions of Need among Service Providers, Yorkshire and Humberside Region.* Yorkshire and Humberside Refugee Support Centre, 2003.

49. Webster A, Rojas-Jaimes C. *The Mental Health Needs of Refugees in Lambeth: results of a consultation exercise with refugee community organizations.* 2000.

50. Civis Trust. *Refugees and Mental Health: a good practice guide for primary care workers.* London: Civis Trust, 2004.

51. Watters C. *Asylum Seekers and Mental Health Care in the UK.* London: Refugee Council, 2002.

52. McColl H, McKenzie K, Bhui K. Mental healthcare of asylum seekers and refugees. *Advances in Psychiatric Treatment* 2008; **14(6)**: 452–9.

53. Gorst-Unsworth C, Goldenberg E. Psychological sequelae of torture and organised violence suffered by refugees from Iraq: trauma-related factors compared with social factors in exile. *British Journal of Psychiatry* 1998; **172**: 90–4.

54. Raj M, Reading J. *A Shattered World: the mental health needs of refugees and newly arrived communities*. London: Migrant and Refugee Communities Forum, CVS Consultants, 2002.

55. National Institute for Clinical Excellence. *Post-Traumatic Stress Disorder (PTSD): the management of PTSD in adults and children in primary and secondary care* (Clinical Guideline 26). London: NICE, 2005, www.nice.org.uk/page.aspx?o=248149 [accessed July 2013].

56. Burnett A, Fassil Y. *Meeting the Health Needs of Refugees and Asylum Seekers in the UK: an information and resource pack for health workers*. London: DH, 2002, http://webarchive. nationalarchives.gov.uk/+/www.dh.gov.uk/en/Publicationsandstatistics/Publications/ PublicationsPolicyAndGuidance/DH_4010199 [accessed July 2013].

57. Feldman R. *Guidance for Commissioning Heath Services for Vulnerable Women*. London: Maternity Action/Women's Health and Equality Consortium, 2012.

58. Haroon S. *The Health Needs of Asylum Seekers*. London: Faculty of Public Health, 2007.

59. Zimmerman C. *Asylum-Seeking Women, Violence & Health: results from a pilot study in Scotland and Belgium*. London: London School of Hygiene and Tropical Medicine, 2009.

60. Momoh C. *Female Genital Mutilation*. Oxford: Radcliffe, 2005.

61. Royal College of Obstetricians and Gynaecologists. *Female Genital Mutilation*. London: RCOG, 2003.

62. Health and Policy Economic Research Unit B. *Meeting the Healthcare Needs of Refugees and Asylum Seekers: a survey of general practitioners*. London: BMA, 2004, www.refugeetoolkit. org.uk/sites/refugeetoolkit/files/imce_user_files/meeting-the-needs-of-asylum-seekers-bma-report.pdf [accessed July 2013].

63. Romero-Ortuño R. Access to health care for illegal immigrants in the EU: should we be concerned? *European Journal of Health Law* 2004; **11**: 245–72.

64. Vernon G. *Belonging and Betrayal*. Amazon, 2013.

65. Vernon G. How to teach trainees about primary care for refugees and asylum seekers. *Education for Primary Care* 2008; **19(4)**: 430–2.

6 Prisoner health issues

Iain Brew

Aim

In this chapter we aim to reach a basic understanding of the organisation and delivery of primary care in the secure environment.

Key learning points

- Understand that there is a large amount of pathology amongst prisoners.

- Be aware that social exclusion begins at a young age.

- Remember that mental health, substance misuse and physical health complaints often coexist.

- Recognise that health improvement can reduce re-offending.

- Understand that secure medicine is a challenging and rewarding specialty for primary care staff.

Introduction

Prisons exist to punish offenders, to satisfy public demands for retribution, to reduce recidivism by removing the most prolific offenders from society (albeit temporarily) and to rehabilitate offenders. Prison populations in the UK have increased dramatically over recent years. In April 2013, the England and Wales prison population was just under 84,000, of which approximately 80,000 were male.[1] Annually, some 140,000 people pass through the prison system with 80% serving six months or less.[2]

Local prisons generally hold remanded and shorter-sentenced prisoners. They also hold prisoners awaiting transfer to 'lifer prisons', for those who have received life sentences, or transfer to 'training' prisons, for those serving more than 12 months (although capacity issues in the overcrowded system mean in reality that local prisons may hold people for much longer periods).

All aspects of prison practice are governed by Prison Service Instructions (PSIs)[3] or Prison Service Orders (PSOs), and health care is no exception. Examples of such Instructions (which may each stretch to over a hundred pages) include PSI 2011-64 Management of Prisoners at Risk of

Harm to Self, to Others and from Others (Safer Custody), PSO 3500 Continuity of Healthcare for Prisoners, PSI 2011-07 Care and Management of Transsexual Prisoners and PSI 2010-45 the Integrated Drug Treatment System (IDTS). It is important for all prison health staff including locums and agency staff to be aware of these orders as they are mandatory and form part of the Service Level Agreements (SLAs) between commissioners and providers of health care in UK prisons.

Imprisoned patients are generally likely to be mistrustful of authority figures, often having suffered social exclusion from a young age. Up to 24% of adult prisoners have been in care[4] at some point during their childhood; many have experienced abuse (29%) or witnessed domestic violence (41%) as a child, particularly where alcohol or drugs were involved. The rate of truancy, school exclusion and resulting illiteracy amongst prisoners is also very high – the reading age of over 40% of all prisoners is quoted as being below 11 years.[5] Such issues lead to these vulnerable people being marginalised by society, where they may 'get in with the wrong crowd', bringing them into conflict with law enforcement agencies and the Criminal Justice System (CJS). Crime – both acquisitive and violent – means that this group understandably attracts less public sympathy and support than they perhaps deserve.

Statistically, prisoners access health care some four to five times more frequently when in prison[5] than the general population. Coexisting illicit drug use, alcohol misuse, mental health problems and the resulting physical health complications make this group particularly challenging in terms of healthcare provision. Smoking rates among prisoners are higher than in matched populations in the community.[6] Low self-esteem and chaotic lifestyles reduce healthcare (and other) appointment attendance rates and can make concordance with recommended treatment difficult to achieve.

Healthcare provision

Before 2004, when the responsibility for commissioning health care in prisons passed from the Home Office to Primary Care Trusts and Health Boards, health care for prisoners lay entirely outside the NHS. Prison health care was largely unregulated, meaning that any registered medical practitioner was permitted under Prison Rules to work as a prison medical officer. As a result of this, standards of patient care varied widely across the country and this variation was compounded by professional isolation.[7]

Over the last nine years, the development of partnership working between the prisons (whose main priority is security) and healthcare providers (whose main priority is patient safety) has generally led to many improvements in health care. Prisoner health is now set firmly within the NHS with Prison Healthcare Performance Indicators coming into line with the Quality and Outcomes Framework (QOF) and the aspiration of offering 'equivalence' in health care is becoming a reality. Some prisons have started the application process for the Quality Practice Award (QPA) to demonstrate the quality of care offered. The new commissioning landscape means that prison health care will be commissioned by NHS England (the National Commissioning Board), and this may present an opportunity to streamline prison health care nationally, bringing increased consistency and cooperation to prison healthcare practice in England.

Management of drug misuse

The majority of patients in the prison setting have substance use issues, with approximately 50–60% addicted to opioid drugs.[8] Poly-drug use is rife: especially crack cocaine, with benzodiazepines and heroin. Additionally, patients' alcohol intake is at often hazardous levels, making their assessment and management extremely complex.

Increasingly, patients admit to the use of newer psychoactive substances including so-called 'legal highs', and these may be clinically relevant too. M-kat or 'miaow-miaow' (4 methylmethcathinone) is a stimulant that can lead to severe depression and suicidality during withdrawal, and this may be relevant in assessing suicide risk in medical reception.

GHB (γ-hydroxybutyrate) and GBL (γ-hydroxybutyrolactone) are intoxicants that can cause euphoria, disinhibition and unconsciousness. The withdrawal may be particularly dangerous for habituated users and deaths have been reported. Detoxification regimes usually require high-dose diazepam (up to 80 mg in several divided doses daily) for γ-aminobutyric acid type A (GABA$_A$) receptors with baclofen to cover γ-aminobutyric acid type B (GABA$_B$) receptor withdrawal.

Ketamine is widely used in certain parts of the UK. Users describe a state of disconnection from reality and out-of-body experiences, colloquially known as 'the k-hole'. Serious damage to the urinary tract may follow extensive ketamine abuse and some patients have required cystectomy and urostomy to manage this. Mexxy (methoxetamine) is used as 'bladder-friendly ketamine', although its undesirable effects such as cerebellar ataxia may last longer than those of ketamine.

The management of substance misuse in the secure setting is broadly similar to that offered in the open community, although prison prescribers are necessarily more paternalistic in their approach. The high numbers and concentration of drug users and dealers along with the age-old practice of trading between prisoners mean less autonomy for prisoner patients as compared with their counterparts outside (see 'Key learning points').

Nurses, drug workers and healthcare officers screen patients on arrival for drug misuse issues. Urine drug screening is mandatory to confirm the presence of the patient's stated substance intake. Most tests offer almost immediate screening results for opioid, methadone, buprenorphine, cocaine, benzodiazepines, amphetamines and cannabis.

Assessment of the patient's withdrawal status and general condition by a suitably trained clinician follows and where necessary a prescription for methadone or buprenorphine is provided. This may be in the form of a detoxification regime, titration against measured withdrawal symptoms, or continuation of confirmed maintenance treatment from an outside prescriber, although guidelines suggest that doses should be split for the first two days in custody for safety reasons. However, patients usually arrive in prison late in the day when pharmacies and drug agencies are closed. It can therefore be difficult or impossible to obtain telephone confirmation of methadone dosage and when the most recent dose was collected or supervised. In these circumstances, to avoid the risk of overdose, substitute prescription doses are titrated from safe levels (between 10–30 ml methadone according to local policy). This may be the first of many sources of conflict with imprisoned patients, making therapeutic alliances more difficult to achieve later on.

Psychosocial intervention is delivered by the Counselling, Assessment, Referral, Advice and Throughcare (CARAT) team, who are the drug workers in English prisons. Agencies were previously commissioned by the Prison Service, so worked separately from healthcare providers, leading to less integrated delivery of care. CARAT teams now work seamlessly with healthcare providers, cooperating on common documentation and providing care in an integrated fashion. The introduction of the Integrated Drug Treatment System (IDTS),[9] an initiative involving all prisons in England, has led to huge improvements in the standard and consistency of care over recent years. The cornerstones of IDTS are:

- increasing availability and quality of care to prisoners
- offering an increased range of treatments
- integrating health care and CARAT work
- improving the continuity of care for patients transferring between prisons.

IDTS has brought enormous investment in staff, training and infrastructure. Areas have been designated for patients to be stabilised in the four weeks following arrival in prison. Cell doors in these areas have been altered to allow access 24 hours a day through a hatch. This not only allows face-to-face assessment and monitoring of vital signs but also means medication can be administered and supervised at any time.

Once stabilised either on maintenance methadone or buprenorphine, prisoners are involved in planning their own care, aiming for reduction in doses and ultimate abstinence if they have reached the end of their opioid careers. IDTS means that patients requiring more long-term maintenance can be treated effectively, but, clearly, maintenance over several years with no end point is untenable. This has been underpinned by the recovery agenda,[10] which encourages abstinence as a primary goal for the majority of users, while acknowledging that there may be a few who will require long-term substitution treatment.

When patients who have successfully completed a detoxification programme are coming up towards release, a further assessment is made of their risk of relapse on regaining their freedom. If clinicians, drug workers and patients feel that the risk of relapse is high, the topic of re-induction of substitute prescribing is considered. In these circumstances, methadone or buprenorphine may be restarted by prison health staff prior to the release date. The rationale of this controversial aspect of treatment is to reduce the craving for opioids on release, reducing the risk of overdose and drug-related death due to loss of tolerance, and encouraging the patient's engagement in treatment back in the community.

Despite the best efforts of prison security departments, smuggling of illicit drugs into prisons is surprisingly common. Large amounts of heroin, buprenorphine tablets and benzodiazepines are brought into prison in the rectums of arriving prisoners (who may even have been paid to get sent to prison by the serving prisoner!). Further supplies may be thrown over the prison walls or brought in by visitors, who may pass drugs when kissing or hugging in the visits area. This continues in spite of searching of visitors, the presence of trained drug detection dogs and CCTV monitoring of the visits hall.

Diversion of prescribed drugs with abuse potential is a problem throughout the prison estate, with patients resorting to the most bizarre means to hoodwink staff who are supervising the administration of medication. Paracetamol tablets have been carved to resemble buprenorphine tablets. These may be switched during supervised dosing and the original sold on the black market. Patients may make use of poor dentition to hide fragments of tablets in cavities or under dental plates. Pouches made of adhesive tape have been found behind the lips of the more expert drug diverter. In extreme cases, prisoners report selling regurgitated methadone to others despite the increasingly widespread availability of prescribed substitute medication. There are clear risks resulting from these behaviours including overdose and the spread of infectious diseases, and this risk management complicates the management of drug users in the secure setting.

....

Learning points

▷ Substance misuse is the most common health threat among prisoners.

▷ Diversion and the black market complicate prescribing.

▷ Harm reduction and stabilisation are goals in prison.

▷ Re-induction of substitute prescribing may be suitable even after detoxification.

....

Management of mental ill-health

There are some startling statistics on mental health problems in the practice of medicine in secure settings. It was estimated in 1998[11] that over 90% of prisoners had one or more of the five psychiatric disorders studied, namely psychosis, neurosis, personality disorder, hazardous drinking and drug dependence. Such patients may not have sought help from healthcare professionals, often living on the fringes of society. If they have been assessed, concordance with management plans may be less than ideal and a lack of stability in housing and other social indices may be significant.

Dual diagnosis (the presence of mental health problems complicated by substance misuse) is very common, and may be a result of patients self-medicating with illicit drugs or alcohol. This behaviour makes patients less likely to remain engaged with their mental health services, potentially leading to a downward spiral, culminating in further criminal activity (often acquisitive crime or violence) and the resulting involvement of the CJS.

Involvement of mental health services at or soon after arrest and assessment of offenders can allow diversion from court rather than imprisoning mentally ill patients. Services vary significantly across England and Wales. The Bradley report (2009)[12] makes a number of recommendations to improve this. That funding and commissioning of health care in police settings should be passed to the NHS at the earliest opportunity is one such recommendation. Others include the provision of mental health awareness training for police, probation staff and the judiciary, and that court diversion services be standardised across the country. Lord Bradley underlined the need for improvements in the management of prisoners suffering from dual diagnosis.

Healthcare officers (prison officers who have received some basic training in health delivery) and general nurses supported by a few mental health nurses have traditionally offered care to mental health patients in the prison setting. However, since 2004 Mental Health In-reach Teams (MHIRTs) managed by Partnership NHS Trusts have worked with primary care providers to improve the care of offenders with mental health problems. Their role has been to care for those offenders suffering 'severe and enduring' mental illness – a working definition has been those prisoners who were on an enhanced level of Care Programme Approach (CPA) in the community. Forensic psychiatrists working with MHIRTs provide secondary care medical input according to the usual model of GP referral. Until recently, there was often a gap in service provision between the GPs and the psychiatrist. Another Bradley recommendation is the provision of robust Primary Mental Health Care teams to work with offenders who are not suffering severe mental illness, but who are in need of more input than can be provided by GPs and general nurse teams.

Suicide and deliberate self-harm in prisoners

Suicide and deliberate self-harm are much more prevalent in the prison population than in the community as a whole. It is widely quoted that the suicide rate in the imprisoned population is between five and ten times the national prevalence rate of approximately 11.8 per 100,000 per year (2011).[13] Risk factors include untreated withdrawal from drugs or alcohol, prisoners on remand for the first time, mental health problems and the imposition of long sentences.

Hanging is the commonest modality of completed suicide and so-called 'safer cells' designed to reduce the number of ligature points are being introduced across the prison estate. Prisoners considered at risk of suicide are located in such cells whenever possible. It remains almost impossible to prevent suicide in the most determined cases, who often give no clue of their intentions before the event.

The screening of new arrivals includes a mental health and suicide risk assessment, and, where significant risk is identified, suicide prevention procedures are opened. Assessment, Care in Custody and Teamwork (ACCT)[14] is what is commonly referred to as a 'suicide watch' and involves brief assessment of the 'pushes' towards suicide and the 'pulls' back from suicide. Following detailed assessment, trained prison or health staff make a care plan to maximise the 'pulls' while minimising the 'pushes' and ensuring regular, meaningful interactions between staff and prisoners. ACCT procedures may be opened by any member of staff who is concerned about a prisoner, and it is mandatory to commence ACCT procedures following any episode of self-harm.

Before ACCT was introduced from 2005, the suicide watch was known as 'F2052SH' – this was mainly an observation tool and consequently not very effective at reducing suicides. Figures from the last two years may suggest a reduction in prisoner suicide – indeed 2011 saw the lowest number of prison suicides (57) since records began. ACCT may be partly responsible for this improvement.

Deliberate self-harm may be a (maladaptive) coping mechanism for some patients in stressful situations; some may use self-harm in a 'goal oriented' fashion in order to derive some secondary gain such as access to an outside hospital or a supply of tobacco. Cutting with razor blades, glass or broken crockery is a common modality of self-harm in both male and female prisoners, but burning with cigarettes and swallowing foreign bodies including razor blades and even cutlery are also well recognised. Behavioural treatments can be very effective at reducing self-harm by introducing alternative coping strategies for these often very damaged and vulnerable people.

Overdose (deliberate or accidental) with prescribed or illicitly acquired medication is a very serious problem in prisons. For this reason, prescribing in the secure setting is more restricted than in the general community. The decision to issue medication 'in possession' (a supply kept by the patient) must be made on the back of a careful risk assessment in each individual case, while not removing all the personal responsibility of individuals by imposing supervised treatments. Various risk assessments are used across the prison estate to enable suitable patients to manage their own medication. Patients in prison will be returning to the wider community and it is important not to foster institutionalisation and over-reliance on healthcare or prison staff.

Management of common physical health problems

Clearly with 140,000 people passing through prisons every year, a wide variety of health problems are likely to present. At any given time, a prison with a roll of 1000 will have several inmates with diabetes and cases of ischaemic heart disease, chronic obstructive pulmonary disease (COPD) and epilepsy. These patients may have defaulted from follow-up at their own general practices (if they are registered at all) and may have been less than compliant with prescribed medication and other lifestyle advice like smoking cessation.

The prison healthcare system affords an excellent opportunity to identify these patients at reception screening and to arrange appropriate investigation, treatment and onward referral as necessary. Assertive outreach by nurses on wings or housing units can allow even the least motivated prisoners the opportunity to receive health education and chronic disease monitoring.

Many patients in prison have led difficult and chaotic lives outside the prison walls. Such patients (if imprisoned for long enough) can be encouraged to attend hospital for expert assessment and management (including surgery) of any ongoing health problems.

By contrast, sending patients to outside hospitals has security impli-cations in terms of escape risk. The majority of prisoners are escorted by prison officers while in hospital, depending upon their security risk assessment. Not only is this costly to the NHS – often over £750 per day – but it can also affect the smooth running of the prison by taking prison staff off the wings. This can adversely affect the other prisoners in the establishment, who may not be able to attend classes or association (time out of their cells for phone calls, showers, etc.).

Complications of intravenous drug use (IVDU) such as deep-vein thrombosis (DVT) and the resulting venous insufficiency and leg ulcers are extremely common amongst prisoners. Doppler ankle-brachial pressure index (ABPI) is an essential skill for nurses to allow four-layer bandaging to allow healing of ulcers in these patients. While it is very sat-isfying to see the healing during a period of incarceration, experienced prison nurses will know the disappointment of seeing a patient return with broken-down skin on their legs if they return to prison having relapsed into old habits on release.

Another common complication of IVDU is hepatitis C. Antibodies are present in approximately 30% of prisoners screened in local prisons. In 2007, the UK prevalence was 0.3–0.7%, primarily among intravenous drug users and certain migrant populations (especially Pakistani and Bangla-deshi where infected blood products and mass vaccination programmes using contaminated needles led in the past to the inadvertent spread of the infection).[15] The treatment of this condition has improved dramatically since the introduction of pegylated interferon alpha-2a and combination treatment with ribavirin, an oral antiviral drug. Sustained viral response (negative viral count at six months post-completion of treatment) can now be achieved in 45–50% of genotype 1 and 75–80% of genotypes 2, 3 and 4.[15] Untreated, some 20% of patients will clear the virus, but 90% of the remainder will end up with cirrhosis after 20–30 years.

The supportive environment of a prison provides an excellent oppor-tunity to treat individuals who are motivated to receive these medica-tions, which can produce unpleasant and potentially dangerous side effects including blood test abnormalities (including thrombocytopenia), malaise, fatigue, depression and weight loss. Several prisons are now offering treatment for hepatitis C to patients under the supervision of hospital consultants in hepatology or infectious diseases. There are some community treatment projects starting around the country and training to accredit GPs to manage hepatitis C in shared-care models. The RCGP has developed the Certificates 1 and 2 in the Detection, Diagnosis and Management of Hepatitis B and C in Primary Care.[16]

Patients in prison regularly present with pain (or supposed pain) resulting from old injuries: fractures and back pain. Complaints of pain from 'nerve damage', leg ulcers and poor dentition come with requests for opioid painkillers, and more recently for neuropathic analgesics such as pregabalin and gabapentin. The latter drugs have sedating effects similar to benzodiazepines, because they stimulate the release of γ-aminobutyric acid (GABA). They also potentiate the effects of opioids (including methadone) and have euphoriant effects making them very appealing to drug users. For this reason, the use of pregabalin is strongly discouraged in the management of drug users. Prison prescribers are regularly faced with dilemmas of treating pain appropriately without adding to the already considerable availability of drugs of abuse. Until recently, there was little formal guidance for prescribers on these difficult issues. This is now being addressed by the RCGP-sponsored training modules[17] and by the increasing collaboration of pharmacists, doctors and nurses through their respective regional Secure Environment Groups.

Safer Prescribing[18] for drugs with abuse potential has been developed by the RCGP working with the Department of Health, the Royal College of Nurses (RCN) and the National Pharmacy Secure Environment Group. It is to be hoped that this guidance will lead to increased consistency between prisons and a reduction in inappropriate prescribing in the secure setting. Further consensus (RCGP, British Pain Society, RCN, Royal Pharmaceutical Society and Department of Health) guidance on the management of chronic pain in secure environments is due to be published in 2013. This will reinforce the importance of physical treatments and the limited role for drug treatment in cases of chronic pain.

Consultation skills for prison GPs

The doctor–patient relationship in the prison setting is necessarily more complex than in the wider community. Patients' statements cannot always be taken at face value, and doctors working in prison must always be alive to the possibility of manipulation at the hands of skilled influencers.

Patients in prison may attempt to obtain drug prescriptions by lying, inventing symptoms (knowing buzz words such as burning or shooting pain and nerve damage) or intimidation and threats of legal action. The more intelligent patient may employ more subtle techniques such as the grooming of doctors' egos, compliments or feigned friendship. Statements such as 'I bet you know all the tricks' and 'I'm not like the others in here' are regularly heard in consultations and should alert the prison doctor to the possibility of manipulation.

When declining inappropriate medication or lifestyle (wearing own clothes etc.) requests, an angry patient is always a possibility. Rarely, doctors have been assaulted by an unhappy prisoner and, although the risk of being taken hostage is small, it is ever present. It is essential that doctors working in the prison setting are aware of basic breakaway techniques (self-defence) and of de-escalation, calming a potentially dangerous situation using both verbal and non-verbal consultation skills.

These skills can also help in the formation of a useful therapeutic relationship where patients feel they can trust their doctors and where information exchange can take place with less scepticism on both sides. Working relationships with drug workers, nurses and doctors can be the first step towards these difficult but vulnerable people reintegrating into society.

Discharge arrangements

Release into the open community is a risky time for prisoners. They are often not registered with a GP, or their registration may have lapsed if they have been in prison for a long time. It is the responsibility of prison health care to assist prisoners with registering on release (PSO 3050 Continuity of healthcare and PSO 2300 Resettlement). At least a week's medication to take out (TTO) is normally issued on release unless there is a danger of overdose. Prescriptions for diazepam, methadone or buprenorphine maintenance are being prescribed on FP10MDA prescriptions in some areas to ensure continuity of care until a community drug team can take over the prescribing. Before the era of opioid substitution prescriptions, drug-related deaths on release were commonplace as patients were likely to relapse into heroin use and overdose having lost their opioid tolerance. There is evidence that the current approach of maintenance prescribing has saved approximately 6–8 such deaths annually in the Leeds area alone (personal communication).

Discharge notification letters should be provided to prisoners to inform their GPs of current medication and health interventions during imprisonment. While most English prisons now use the computerised record 'SystmOne', current confidentiality rules mean that released prisoners must ask their GPs to request full records with written consent. This means in practice that GPs very often do not receive any information about their patients' health care during periods of imprisonment. Changes in GP registration legislation are expected over the coming years to remedy this deficiency, and it is hoped that the prison SystmOne records will be linked to the NHS spine at some point.

....

Learning points

▷ Patients are normally released with a week's TTO medication.

▷ Release on substitute opioids saves lives.

▷ GP registration is often a problem for prisoners.

▷ Receiving GPs can and should request prison health records with patient consent.

....

Case scenario

Jimmy is an emaciated 32-year-old heroin user who has been remanded in custody for his twenty-third shoplifting charge. He says that he injects £50 worth of heroin daily and smokes crack cocaine worth £30 daily. Until four months ago, he was in treatment with a community drug team at the local no fixed abode (NFA) practice, but he stopped attending because he knew the police were looking for him. He has a painful leg ulcer due to venous insufficiency following a DVT caused by groin injecting. He thinks he may have hepatitis C from sharing needles. You see him in reception on a Friday night. He is suffering chills and is nauseated due to his withdrawal symptoms. He last injected yesterday.

1 What immediate steps will you take to ensure Jimmy's safety?

2 What issues will you consider in forming your care plan for Jimmy?

3 How will you try to ensure continuity of care for this complex case?

4 What factors might prevent Jimmy remaining in treatment?

....

Two weeks later, Jimmy is stable on a 40 ml daily dose of methadone. He thanks you for being so helpful and says that you are the best doctor he has ever met. He looks much better than when you met him in reception and is gaining weight well. He goes on to request painkillers for his leg ulcer. He says that pregabalin has worked for him before.

5 What does Jimmy's behaviour make you consider?

6 How will you manage his request?

7 What alternatives could you offer?

....

You review Jimmy after a further two weeks. He says that his court appearance led to a three-month sentence, so he will be released in another two weeks. (Having served half the sentence, he will be on licence for the remaining six weeks.) His ulcer is healing with four-layer bandaging and he is stable on 40 ml of methadone daily.

8 How will you plan for Jimmy's release into the community?

9 What will you mention on his discharge letter for his GP?

10 How many factors in Jimmy's history make him likely to return to prison?

....

Sample answers

1 Assess withdrawal symptoms, confirm presence of drugs on urine drug screening and prescribe opioid substitute such as methadone 10–20 ml. ('Start low and go slow' when titrating the dose.) Check for DVT and prescribe oral anticoagulants (such as rivaroxaban) or low molecular weight heparin until Doppler scan organised. Consider alcohol or benzodiazepine withdrawal. Consider suicide risk: ? mental health assessment.
....

2 Will Jimmy engage with drug services again? Care plan for leg ulcer? Doppler ABPI and four-layer bandaging. Is he remanded or sentenced? Is it feasible to treat his hepatitis?
....

3 Communication (with patient's consent) between outside agency and GP who were treating him before and prison services. Communication with CARAT workers, nurses and prison staff.
....

4 Jimmy may be upset with the doctor's prescribing – patients often want more medication than safety allows. He may have brought drugs into prison in his rectum or may prefer to continue using drugs illicitly in the prison.
....

5 Praise and over-familiarity may be techniques of manipulation. Jimmy may be massaging your ego to ensure you are more sympathetic to his requests. The prescriber must always be alert to this possibility.
....

6 First, it is important to treat the root of the problem by arranging an assessment for four-layer bandaging to heal the ulcers. Venous insufficiency is the most likely cause of the ulcers in this context. Managing infection (not colonisation) is important and a vascular referral may be necessary. It is essential that the patient understands these issues. An explanation of why pregabalin is not routinely prescribed (because of widespread abuse in prison) is important.
....

101

7 It is important to manage infection in ulcers, which may exacerbate pain. Appropriate assessment and dressing will help to manage pain. Simple analgesia should be offered first using some sort of pain ladder. Opioids should be avoided if possible. Low-dose amitriptyline may be helpful. Lidocaine patches applied topically to unbroken skin near the area of pain are being used to manage genuine neuropathic pain.

8 Communication with outside prescribers is vital to ensure a seamless transfer of care. Any gap between release and outside appointments may need to be covered by the prison prescriber, possible using an FP10MDA (prescription for instalment prescribing). Jimmy may need help in registering with a GP – this is now the responsibility of the releasing prison healthcare department.

9 Investigation results and treatment (e.g. of the leg ulcer) need to be shared with the GP. Any plans for treating hepatitis C or other hospital referrals should be included in discharge letters. Dosage of prescribed drugs (especially if benzodiazepine reduction has been commenced) is vital as prisoners often present inaccurate accounts of their prescribed medication on release from prison.

10 Jimmy has a long history of recidivism and recent chaotic drug use. His short sentence has not given him enough time to address his drug use fully, meaning he may not be motivated to remain in treatment with his community drug treatment service. His physical health problems have not been dealt with fully due to his short sentence, making it likely that he will be in pain from leg ulcers and worried about his hepatitis. Both of these concerns place him at higher risk of relapse into drug misuse. It is unlikely that Jimmy has sorted out his housing issue; homelessness is a huge risk factor for re-offending.

Further reading

- Department of Health, HM Prison Service. *Prison Health Handbook*. London: DH, HM Prison Service, 2003.

- Department of Health (England) and the devolved administrations. *Drug Misuse and Dependence: UK guidelines on clinical management*. London: DH (England), the Scottish Government, Welsh Assembly Government and Northern Ireland Executive, 2007.

- Marteau D, Farrell M. Clinical management of substance misuse in prisons. In C Gerada (ed.). *RCGP Guide to the Management of Substance Misuse in Primary Care*. London: RCGP, 2005, pp. 333–44.

- RCGP Secure Environments Group. *Safer Prescribing in Prisons: guidance for clinicians.* Nottingham: Nottinghamshire Healthcare, 2011, www.rcgp.org.uk/news/2011/november/ new-guidance-on-prison-prescribing.aspx [accessed July 2013].

References

1. Ministry of Justice Weekly Prison Population Bulletin, 11 April 2013.

2. Department of Health, HM Prison Service. *Prison Health Handbook.* London: DH, HM Prison Service, 2003.

3. Prison Service Instructions (PSIs), www.justice.gov.uk/offenders/psis [accessed July 2013].

4. Williams K, Papadopoulou V, Booth N. *Prisoners' Childhood and Family Backgrounds: results from the Surveying Prisoner Crime Reduction (SPCR) longitudinal cohort study of prisoners.* Ministry of Justice Analytical Services, 2012.

5. Marshall T, Simpson S, Stevens A. *Health Care in Prisons: a health care needs assessment.* Birmingham. University of Birmingham, 2000.

6. Prison Service Instruction 09/2007. Smoke Free Legislation – Prison Service Application. HM Prison Service. 2007.

7. Joint Prison Service and National Health Service Executive Working Group. *The Future Organisation of Prison Health Care.* London: DH, 1999.

8. Marteau D, Farrell M. Clinical management of substance misuse in prisons. In C Gerada (ed.). *RCGP Guide to the Management of Substance Misuse in Primary Care.* London. RCGP, 2005, pp. 333–44.

9. Integrated Drug Treatment System, www.justice.gov.uk/downloads/offenders/psipso/psi-2010/psi_2010_45_IDTS.doc [accessed July 2013].

10. Singleton N. *Psychiatric Morbidity among Prisoners in England and Wales: the report of a survey carried out in 1997 by Social Survey Division of the Office of National Statistics on behalf of the Department of Health.* London: TSO, 1998.

11. National Treatment Agency. *Commissioning for Recovery. Drug treatment, reintegration and recovery in the community and prisons: a guide for drug partnerships.* London: NTA, 2010, www.nta.nhs.uk/ uploads/commissioning_for_recovery_january_2010.pdf [accessed July 2013].

12. Bradley K. *The Bradley Report: Lord Bradley's review of people with mental health problems or learning disabilities in the Criminal Justice System.* London: DH, 2009.

13. Office for National Statistics. Statistical bulletin: Suicides in the United Kingdom. 2011.

14. HM Prison Service. PSI 2011-64 Management of prisoners at risk of harm to self, to others and from others (Safer Custody). 2012.

15. Costella A. *Hepatitis C in the UK 2008.* London: Health Protection Agency Centre for Infections, 2008.

16. RCGP Certificate in the Detection, Diagnosis and Management of Hepatitis B and C in Primary Care Part 1, www.rcgp.org.uk/courses-and-events/substance-misuse-and-associated-health/ [accessed July 2013].

17. MSc Healthcare in Secure Environments, www.lincoln.ac.uk/home/course/hltrltms/ [accessed July 2013].

18. RCGP Secure Environments Group. *Safer Prescribing in Prisons: guidance for clinicians.* Nottingham: Nottinghamshire Healthcare, 2011, www.rcgp.org.uk/news/2011/november/ new-guidance-on-prison-prescribing.aspx [accessed July 2013].

7

Caring for older people
in primary care

Louise Robinson

Aim

As people age, changes in personal and professional circumstances lead to older people becoming socially isolated and hence marginalised. Children growing up and moving away, retirement, and loss of family and friends due to illness and death can considerably reduce older peoples' social networks. Social isolation has proven impacts on an older person's health and wellbeing both physically and mentally. One particular group of older people who face considerable social stigma and often a loss of social contacts are those with dementia. People living with dementia and their families also face challenges in accessing appropriate and timely care and support. The aim of this chapter is to highlight the inequalities in care received by one particularly disadvantaged group of older people, those living with dementia. The chapter gives an overview of the epidemiology of dementia, the clinical presentation and subsequent investigation, and the key areas of primary care management of this illness including holistic care, ethical and legal issues, carer support, symptom management and end-of-life care.

Key learning points

- Understand how dementia presents in primary care, including relevant epidemiology.

- Assess and investigate a person with suspected dementia.

- Adopt a holistic approach to the primary care management of people with dementia and understand when to refer to secondary care and community services.

- Know the legal and ethical issues relevant to the care of people with dementia.

- Identify when to use pharmacological and non-pharmacological managements.

Introduction

Europe is rapidly ageing; life expectancy is increasing by two years every decade. Current estimates predict that the proportion of people over 65 years will increase from 20% in 2000 to 35% in 2050,[1] generating a ratio of 4.3 persons over 80 years for every child in the population. Those aged 85 and over, *the oldest old*, are now the fastest growing sector of the population. In the UK, improving the health of our older people is a key policy area;[2,3] however, we can expect an increase in age-related illnesses, such as dementia, osteoarthritis and stroke. This will present considerable challenges for healthcare providers in the UK, particularly for primary care, with policy that increasingly stipulates that care for older people, and for those with long-term conditions, should be delivered as close to their homes as possible.[4]

In terms of health care, one particularly disadvantaged group of older people are those living with dementia. Evidence has consistently revealed that they receive suboptimal care in many areas including unacceptable delays in diagnosis, inappropriate medication, such as the prescription of antipsychotic drugs for behavioural problems, and poor-quality end-of-life care.[5] This chapter focuses on the care of people with dementia to highlight how, as GPs, we can reduce such inequalities of care and ensure they receive the best possible care within primary care.

Dementia: impact and burden

Dementia is one of the main causes of disability in later life; in terms of global burden of disease, it contributes 11.2% of all years lived with disability, higher than stroke (9.5%), musculoskeletal disorders (8.9%), heart disease (5%) and cancer (2.4%). In the UK, there are currently around 700,000 people with dementia but this is estimated to rise to 1.7 million by 2050.[6] The total costs of caring for people with dementia in the UK have been estimated at around £17 billion per year, more than heart disease (£4 billion), stroke (£3 billion) and cancer (£2 billion).[6] Currently around two-thirds of people with dementia live in private households, with the majority of their care provided by family supporters (informal carers) and primary and community care teams.

The GP curriculum and dementia

Within primary care, GPs admit to difficulties in both the diagnosis and management of dementia.[7] Statement 3.05 of the GP curriculum (*Care of Older Adults*) calls for an understanding of the special features of psychiatric disease in old age, including an appreciation of the features of dementia.[8] Specifically GPs must be able to assess brain function and have knowledge of:

- the prevalence and incidence of disease, including dementia, in the elderly population

- the relevant questions in the history and items in the physical examination to the problem presented

- the patient's relevant context, including family and social factors

- the structure of the local and national healthcare system, and the role of primary care within the wider NHS, including knowledge of when to refer to secondary care services

- the inter-relationships between health and social care

- the legal issues that may arise

- the special features associated with drug treatment of dementia.

This chapter will address these key areas.

Raising awareness of dementia in primary care

In England, the National Dementia Strategy[9] identifies 17 objectives to improve the quality of dementia care, including raising both public and professional awareness of dementia (objective 1) and facilitating earlier and more timely diagnosis (objective 2).

One in 14 people aged over 65 years has a form of dementia, rising to one in six of those over 85. A GP with an average list size of 2000 patients, in an area of average demography, will have about 15 patients with dementia of any form. Currently, a GP will meet one or two new cases per year although both incidence and prevalence figures will increase as our population ages. In the UK, the National Quality and Outcomes Framework requires all GP practices to maintain a dementia register. All patients on the register must receive an annual care review; however, the format and content of this review has not been standardised, which will inevitably lead to inequalities within primary care.

Evidence currently shows that around half the people with dementia in primary care have not received a formal diagnosis.[5] In the UK, the time from a patient first presenting with symptoms of dementia to formally receiving a diagnosis is on average 18 months but can take up to four years.[10] A number of reasons for such diagnostic delays have been suggested: a sense by some GPs that nothing can be done; a reluctance by both patients and carers to acknowledge their difficulties, often due to an assumption it is all part of 'normal ageing'; and the well-documented fear and stigma that exist around dementia. Although for some patients receiving a diagnosis of dementia may be distressing, the international consensus is that overall earlier diagnosis of dementia is beneficial, allowing the provision of psychological support, legal and financial advice, and an opportunity for future care planning.[11,12]

Age is the biggest single risk factor for dementia; vascular risk factors play a role in both vascular and mixed dementia, and, as shown by new research, increasingly in Alzheimer's disease too. In the UK, screening for

> ## Box 7.1 **Types of dementias**
>
> ### Alzheimer's disease (AD)
>
> - Most common form (~60% of all dementias).
> - Gradual onset.
> - Early symptoms: memory loss.
> - Late symptoms: language difficulties, behavioural problems such as aggression, wandering.
>
> ### Vascular dementia
>
> - With mixed dementia (AD and vascular), accounts for ~27% of all dementias.
> - Often abrupt onset; may be related to stroke or brain haemorrhage.
> - Fluctuating course with stepwise deterioration.
>
> ### Dementia with Lewy bodies
>
> - Characteristic picture: fluctuating cognitive impairment, visual hallucinations, spontaneous Parkinsonism.
> - Memory relatively spared: cognitive loss related to attention and visuospatial problems.
>
> ### Rare dementias
>
> - These include frontal lobe dementia and Huntington's disease.

dementia is not currently recommended; a pre-dementia stage termed 'mild cognitive impairment' (MCI) has been identified where definite memory changes are present but do not impair an individual's functional ability to lead a normal life. However, the clinical use of the label MCI remains controversial, as research has shown that only around one-fifth of such people go on to develop dementia.

Diagnosis of dementia: primary care management and the role of secondary care

The term dementia relates to a number of different dementia syndromes (see Box 7.1). However, a common range of symptoms can be observed in the different stages of the illness (see Box 7.2). In the early stages, there may be obvious memory difficulties, invariably short-term memory loss, such as forgetting the names of objects and places, and also

Box 7.2 **Presentation and investigation of possible dementia in primary care**

Suspicious symptoms

- Early stage (MMSE score >21): memory loss; poor judgement and reasoning; confusion; mood disturbance; personality changes.

- Middle stage (MMSE score ≤20): worsening memory problems; speech and communication difficulties; problems with activities of daily living; behavioural and psychological symptoms; physical injuries and safety hazards.

- Late stage: swallowing difficulties; malnutrition; incontinence; frailty and immobility.

Investigations in primary care in early and middle stages of dementia

- Cognitive function tests.

- Blood tests: full blood count; urea and electrolytes; thyroid tests; mid-stream urine; ECG and chest X-ray.

Differential diagnosis

Depression, hypothyroidism, vitamin B_{12} deficiency, alcohol problems, or rarely brain tumour or normal-pressure hydrocephalus.

the inability to perform activities of daily living in the correct sequence. Communication difficulties and changes in personality and mood may also ensue, leading GPs to make an initial inaccurate diagnosis of depression, although depression may coexist alongside dementia.

As the illness progresses, the patient with dementia may experience greater difficulties with independent living and may be at risk in terms of his or her personal safety through leaving gas/electricity/bath taps on. Non-cognitive symptoms are particularly distressing for families; these are usually referred to as behavioural and psychological symptoms of dementia (BPSD). Between 20–60% of people with dementia will experience BPSD at some time, particularly in the middle and later stages of the illness. BPSD encompasses a range of symptoms from agitation through to wandering and getting lost. The risks from such behaviour are often not as great as assumed by carers but can lead them to curtail the activities of a patient with dementia.[13]

In the later stages of dementia, communication can be lost entirely and the person may no longer recognise loved ones or may mistake them for someone else: a particularly distressing symptom for families. Swallowing difficulties are common and poor nutrition can lead to recurrent infections such as pneumonia or urinary tract infections, which may eventually be fatal.

Recognising the early signs of dementia is often not easy due to the insidious presentation of the illness and the mirroring of the cognitive and memory changes with those of normal ageing. Individuals and their families may successfully hide their cognitive symptoms by restricting their usual routine and allowing family members to take over tasks (see case scenario 1). Family carers often present their concerns to the GP before the patient him or herself attends.[10] Such complex third-party (or triadic) consultations involving family members can be challenging as both the patient with dementia and his or her carer will have issues to address. Anxieties may also be raised by professionals through missed hospital appointments, unpaid bills and prescribing problems.[10]

....

Case scenario 1

A 77-year-old woman, Mrs S, attends the GP surgery with her son. She had been widowed two years ago. Her son was concerned as he felt she had become more forgetful over the last year. Also he had discovered a cupboard full of unused medications for her blood pressure and heart disease; recently he had noticed her breathing was much worse. The woman denied that her physical health was a problem to her, although admitted that she had become more tired recently and has stopped going to the large supermarket to get her shopping, as it was too far away. She preferred to visit the corner shop while her family now bought her main weekly shopping. Since her husband's death, her son had arranged for most of her bills to be paid by direct debit.

....

In the UK, guidelines on dementia care provide a clear pathway for the detection and referral of people with a suspected dementia.[11] Notwithstanding such clarity, a recent UK report on dementia highlighted suboptimal performance in this area, with the reported time to diagnosis in the UK twice that of some other European countries.[5] GPs in the UK appear to carry out 'watchful waiting' rather than referring at an early stage.[10] In case scenario 1, the GP should take a detailed history from both the patient and accompanying carer, carry out a physical examination and perform some essential investigations (see Box 7.2 on p. 109).[11] Mrs S should be referred for a specialist secondary care assessment, preferably by an old-age psychiatrist, who will instigate detailed neuro-cognitive assessment and, if available, a brain scan to confirm the diagnosis and possibly identify the dementia subtype. The key features of these different subtypes are highlighted in Box 7.1 (see p. 108). Memory clinics provide specialist centres that allow GPs to facilitate an early multidisciplinary assessment of memory problems.[12]

Use of cognitive function tests in primary care

Tests are available for use in the community to make an initial assessment of a patient's cognitive function.[11] The most commonly used tool is the Mini-Mental State Examination (MMSE),[15] which is scored out of 30. A score of <24 is suggestive of dementia; however, it is important to note that, in dementia, a person's functional ability may not be reflected by the MMSE (see Box 7.2 on p. 109). The MMSE can take up to 20 minutes to complete and is now under copyright, leading to issues over its use within the NHS. In general practice, an abbreviated MMSE or other brief cognitive tests, such as the General Practitioner Assessment of Cognition (GPCOG)[16] or 6-Item Cognitive Impairment Test (6-CIT), may be used.[17] All three of these tests are recommended in the NICE guidance on dementia care.[11] In addition, the Clock Drawing Test may be added; here, the patient is asked to draw a clock, number it accurately and add a specified time correctly.[18] The GPCOG is estimated to take 6–7 minutes to complete (four minutes for the patient, three minutes for the carer); such shorter tests may be more relevant for general practice.[19] In the UK, national guidance on how practically to assess cognition has just been released via the Alzheimer's Society.[20]

Disclosure of a diagnosis of dementia: saying the 'D' word

Notwithstanding their expertise in the area of communication skills, GPs appear reluctant to discuss a diagnosis of dementia, a hesitancy that is not seen with other long-term conditions, for example cancer, and carers are more frequently informed of the diagnosis than the person with the illness.[21] How can we improve upon our current performance? In the UK, the National Dementia Strategy for England will hopefully begin to address the desperate need to raise awareness of this condition. In general, however, we need to overcome our own professional demons and be able to talk openly and sensitively about dementia. It would appear that as GPs we need training and support to enable us to feel sufficiently comfortable to say the 'D' word ourselves before we can talk openly to our patients![22]

Support and information

The GP is in a key position to provide much-needed support and advice to a patient and his or her family when the patient discovers he or she has dementia. The Alzheimer's Society has a wide range of information resources and practical support, including day care and befriending services, for people living with all types of dementia (www.alzheimers. org.uk). Signposting families to their local branch of the Society, as well as discussing the role of social services and potential respite services, should be integrated into the primary care consultation.[23]

Listening to a patient's experiences, issues and concerns should be an essential part of the GP consultation. Providing simple cognitive and emotional coping strategies within the primary care consultation has also been shown to be of benefit for both the patient and his or her family. In addition, more specialist psychological therapies, such as Cognitive Behavioural Therapy, if available, have also been shown to help people with dementia.[23] Strategies such as emphasising the positive aspects of his or her life (reframing), reformulating catastrophic thoughts (reality orientation) and the use of memory enhancement strategies and tools are beneficial. However, such expertise may not be readily available to all primary care teams and more widespread distribution of such specialist services is urgently needed.

Long-term holistic care for people with dementia in primary care

On average, people with dementia live around five years from the emergence of their symptoms. For people with vascular dementia, risk factors, such as blood pressure control and lipid management, should be closely monitored in the early and moderate stages of the disease. However, evidence is increasingly emerging that such risk factors may also play a role in Alzheimer's dementia. In general though, there is consistent evidence that the standard of dementia care in the UK is in urgent need of improvement, with frequent failure to deliver services in a timely, integrated or cost-effective manner.[5] As yet no medical intervention exists that can alter the disease process and it has been suggested that a palliative care approach be adopted from the point of diagnosis.[24,25]

More recently, the concept of *supportive care* has been suggested, which acknowledges a holistic approach throughout the dementia care pathway.[26] Supportive care is defined as the multidisciplinary holistic care of patients and their families from the time around diagnosis, through treatments aimed at cure or prolonging life, and into the phase currently acknowledged as palliative care. It involves recognising and caring for the side effects of active therapies as well as patients' co-morbidities and psychological, social and spiritual concerns. It also values the role of family carers and helps them in supporting the patient, as well as attending to their special needs.[27]

From the GP's perspective, the long-term care of people with dementia requires the same systematic approach as the management of other long-term conditions, namely:

- systematic follow-up of both the person with dementia and his or her main carer, if the latter is also a patient in the GP practice

- emotional and psychosocial support to both the person with dementia and his or her carer

- symptom control including BPSD management

- Advance Care Planning (ACP) and end-of-life care.

Shared care of people with dementia

Acetylcholinesterase inhibitors (donepezil, galantamine, rivastigmine) are the mainstay of treatment in the UK for Alzheimer's disease. Guidance on the prescribing of these drugs has been developed.[28] Memantine, a glutamatergic partial antagonist, was originally licensed for moderately severe to severe Alzheimer's disease, but in the UK its use is restricted to people with moderate to severe dementia who are participating in clinical trials.[28] Apart from rivastigmine, no other drugs are currently licensed for the symptomatic treatment of people with dementias other than Alzheimer's. In the UK, family doctors are not allowed to initiate such drug treatments; only specialists in the care of people with dementia can do so. Since 2004, all English Primary Care Organisations have been required by the National Service Framework for Older People to have a shared-care protocol in place to facilitate shared-care management, between primary and secondary care, of patients who continue on these drugs.[29]

Caring for the carers of people with dementia

In general two-thirds of people with dementia live independently in the community while one-third live in care homes. In the UK around half a million informal carers provide the mainstay of community support and are often the experts in the care needs of the person with dementia.[6] However, carers of people with dementia are more likely to experience depressed mood, to report a higher 'burden' and to have worse physical health, compared with carers of people with other long-term conditions.[30] Depressed mood in the carer is one of the factors that influence the move of the person with dementia to residential care. Unfortunately there is some evidence that carers feel reluctant to seek professional help in such circumstances and only when at a crisis.[31]

In dementia, carers may grieve or experience loss as their relative loses functional and cognitive abilities, and companionship, affection and intimacy are affected. The satisfaction carers experience from caring, the support they receive and their ability to seek help when needed influence how the carers cope. GPs and the primary care team are well placed to monitor the physical and mental wellbeing of carers, to signpost them to sources of information and practical support, and to provide, or refer them for, additional psychological support. Facilitating positive coping strategies and problem-solving behaviour in carers appear to be effective and reduce depression.[23,30]

Management of behavioural and psychological symptoms in dementia

Between 20–60% of people with dementia will experience BPSD at some time, particularly in the middle and later stages. While the risks, such as wandering and getting lost, from such behaviour are often not as high as families fear,[13] they can lead to high levels of carer stress, curtailment of the activities of the person with dementia and may be the critical factor that leads to a care home move.

Non-pharmacological management for such symptoms is initially recommended but this may be difficult to achieve in the community.[11] There is little high-quality evidence for the clinical and cost-effectiveness of such treatments, although research is emerging that illustrates the potential of exercise, behavioural interventions and educational interventions for carers and care home staff.[11] Currently, it is all too easy within primary care to prescribe medication for such symptoms, often due to a lack of availability of specialist psychological services. Between 20–50% of people with dementia in care homes in the UK receive antipsychotic medication,[32] despite widespread concerns over the hazards of using these drugs in dementia;[33] they can be safely withdrawn even in people with dementia who have taken them for prolonged periods.[34]

....

Case scenario 2

Mr and Mrs W attend the GP surgery. Mrs W has had Alzheimer's disease for three years and her last MMSE was 17. Mr W singlehandedly cares for her at home; their only son lives 200 miles away. Current medical input is via the GP and a community psychiatric nurse who visits monthly. Mrs W attends the day centre, often reluctantly, for one day a week.

Mr W reports that his wife has started to wander at night. This is disturbing his sleep and he is feeling more exhausted. On several occasions he has found her in the garden. Mr W wants to continue caring for his wife at home and does not wish her to go to hospital unnecessarily. Mrs W becomes distressed and tearful at this point in the consultation, muttering she wants to be left alone at home.

Advice from the National Institute for Health and Care Excellence provides a helpful framework for GPs to manage BPSD;[11] a typical example is provided in case scenario 2. In this instance, a thorough assessment by the GP is essential to exclude treatable causes such as a urine or chest infection. Non-pharmacological approaches should be used where possible and, if available, referral to specialist nurses, or psychological therapists, will provide support and advice for the family or care home staff. If the distressing behaviours continue, a variety of drug options can be tried depending on the nature and severity of the behaviour (see Box 7.3).[35] Prescribing antipsychotic drugs should be time-limited and only reserved for severe and distressing symptoms after careful assessment of the risks and benefits of their use. National guidance via the UK Alzheimer's Society is now available regarding the optimal management of behavioural problems in dementia.[36]

Advance Care Planning

ACP is a process of discussion between a patient and professional carer, and sometimes family carers. Potential outcomes include: 1) an 'advance statement' – patient preferences for future care; 2) an 'advance

---

Box 7.3 Pharmacological treatments for agitation and behavioural problems in dementia (daily doses) care

Mild agitation

Options include:

- trazodone (50–300 mg)

- selective serotonin reuptake inhibitors, e.g. citalopram (10–20 mg)

- clomethiazole, 1–3 capsules (5–15 ml liquid).

Sodium valproate and carbamazepine may also be considered.

Moderate – severe agitation and psychotic symptoms

- Quetiapine (25–200 mg).

- Risperidone (0.5–2 mg).

- Olanzapine (2.5–10 mg).

Severe behavioural problems

- Haloperidol (0.5–4 mg) (but should be time-limited).

---

directive' or living will – informed consent to refuse certain treatment in specific circumstances, if loss of mental capacity ensues; and 3) a Lasting Power of Attorney, where a person names another to act on his or her behalf, should he or she lose capacity to consent, in areas of the person's health and/or financial welfare. 2) and 3) are legally binding documents. Guidance on how to approach ACP exists for both patients and professionals, but there still appears to be a knowledge transfer gap into practice.[37-39] Notwithstanding this advice, evidence regarding the effectiveness of ACP in influencing health care and patient choice is limited.[40]

In dementia, guidance recommends that ACP discussions should be discussed with the person while he or she still has capacity.[11] In case scenario 2 the GP has an opportunity for discussion with both the patient with dementia and her carer, and document their wishes and preferences for future care, if this has not already been done. In addition, by arranging a separate appointment to see Mr W, perhaps while his wife is at the day centre, the GP could assess Mr W's physical and mental health, discuss his needs as a carer in more detail and also broach legal and financial issues, like power of attorney.

Assessment of capacity and the Mental Capacity Act

A significant number of the oldest old, especially those in nursing homes, will have cognitive impairment, even if a formal diagnosis of dementia has not been made. In the UK, the Mental Capacity Act (Adults with Incapacity Act in Scotland) stipulates that people must be assumed to have mental capacity regardless of age, appearance or behaviour.[41] However, if capacity has been lost, specific guidance must be sought and an appropriate consultee, usually the next of kin or immediate carer, identified who will be then responsible for issues of consent. Assessment of capacity in practice is a complex and difficult area for GPs and advice may be needed from colleagues in old-age psychiatry. Protocols or clinical pathways can be used to assess the key areas that define capacity, namely the older person's ability to understand, retain and use the information to make a decision and the ability to communicate that decision.

End-of-life care

Caring for people with advanced dementia, particularly with respect to symptom management, is challenging due to the severe communication problems that are often present.[25] Ascertaining whether their distress is due to pain, depression or other symptoms is difficult, especially for health professionals who do not know the patient well. A detailed history from family, carers or experienced care home staff may help clarify the situation and facilitate appropriate treatment. Predicting how long a person with advanced dementia may live is also extremely difficult and can be inaccurate even using defined prognostic criteria. Guidance has been produced to help identify patients nearing the last 6–12 months of life and thus trigger better assessment and planning of care related to their needs. For patients with dementia it includes the 'surprise question' ('Would you, as a health professional, be surprised if this patient died within the next year?'), clinical indicators of dementia, and markers of physical decline.[42] GPs need to recognise when treatment or intervention is unnecessary and when extra care or support is needed.

Evidence has shown that only 2% of people with dementia die in a hospice; the GP should consider a referral to his or her community palliative care team or advice and support on the care of the patient dying with dementia sooner rather than later. However, the majority of people with advanced dementia spend the last year of their life in a care home. GPs and community nurses have frequent contact with care homes but, despite this, the quality of care received by older people in nursing homes is variable. There is a need to develop structured, proactive care, with shared working and better communication between primary and care home staff.[26] ACP has an important role in influencing the care received by older people in nursing homes and, although there is evidence that unnecessary hospital admissions can be reduced, a better understanding of how to translate theory into practice in this area is urgently needed.[43] Using an end-of-life care pathway provides a structured approach to care for the person with dementia in the last few days of life.[42,44] The pathway supports nursing and care staff in the community in the delivery of a high standard of end-of-life care. However, identification of end-stage dementia is difficult, and any end-of-life pathway needs to accommodate that difficulty.

Although the majority of people with dementia die in care homes, for most older people their preferred place of death would be their own homes. People with dementia have the right to make such a choice and, as healthcare professionals, it is imperative that we try to ensure, as much as possible, that their choices are fulfilled. In the UK, it is heartening to see an increasing number of local schemes to facilitate people with dementia dying at home.[45,46] Although further evaluation is needed to evaluate such innovative projects,[46] it is at least a step in the right direction towards ensuring people with dementia are no longer doubly disadvantaged in both how they live and how they die with their illness.

Applied Knowledge Test (AKT) questions: drugs for dementia

1 Which is the **SINGLE MOST** appropriate statement in relation to cholinesterase inhibitor symptom-modifying drugs for dementia? *Select ONE option only.*

a Help all types of dementia

b Are licensed for mild cognitive impairment

c May be initiated by the GP

d Are of similar efficacy

e Help all Alzheimer's sufferers to some extent

2 Which is the **SINGLE LEAST** appropriate management option when considering a 75-year-old woman with moderate dementia presenting with a sudden onset of general confusion and agitated behaviour at night? *Select ONE option only.*

a Admit to hospital for assessment

b Ensure a mid-stream urine specimen is collected and sent

c Prescribe an antipsychotic drug such as haloperidol

d Arrange a domiciliary assessment by her consultant

e Request the community psychiatric nurse to visit

Answers: **1 = d | 2 = b**

Useful resources

- Alzheimer's Society
Devon House, 58 St Katharine's Way, London E1W 1JX
Email: enquiries@alzheimers.org.uk | Website: www.alzheimers.org.uk

- Carers Trust
32–36 Loman Street, London SE1 0EH
Email: info@carers.org | Website: www.carers.org

References

1. World Health Organization. *Global Burden of Dementia in the Year 2000*. Geneva: WHO, 2003, www.who.int/entity/healthinfo/statistics/bod_dementia.pdf [accessed July 2013].

2. Department of Health. *NHS R&D Strategic Review: ageing and age-associated disease and disability*. Report of Topic Working Group. London: DH, 1999.

3. Department of Health. *National Service Framework for Older People*. London: DH, 2001.

4. Department of Health. *Our Health, Our Care, Our Say: a new direction for community services. Health and social care working together in partnership*. London: DH, 2006, www.official-documents.gov.uk/document/cm67/6737/6737.pdf [accessed July 2013].

5. National Audit Office. *Improving Services and Support for People with Dementia*. London: TSO, 2007.

6. Alzheimer's Society. *Dementia UK: the full report*. London: Alzheimer's Society, 2007.

7. Turner S, Illiffe S, Downs M, *et al*. General practitioners' knowledge, confidence and attitudes in the diagnosis and management of dementia. *Age and Ageing* 2004; **33(5)**: 461–7.

8. Royal College of General Practitioners. *Care of Older Adults* (Curriculum Statement 3.05). London: RCGP, 2013.

9. Department of Health. *Living Well with Dementia: a national dementia strategy*. London: DH, 2009, www.gov.uk/government/publications/living-well-with-dementia-a-national-dementia-strategy [accessed July 2013].

10. Bamford C, Eccles M, Steen N, *et al*. Can primary care record review facilitate earlier diagnosis of dementia? *Family Practice* 2007; **24(2)**: 108–16.

11. National Institute for Health and Clinical Excellence, Social Care Institute for Excellence. *Dementia: supporting people with dementia and their carers in health and social care*. London: NICE, SCIE, 2006.

12. Waldemar G, Phung KTT, Burns A, *et al*. Access to diagnostic evaluation and treatment for dementia in Europe. *International Journal of Geriatric Psychiatry* 2007; **22(1)**: 47–54.

13. Robinson L, Hutchings D, Corner L, *et al*. Balancing rights and risks – conflicting perspectives in the management of wandering in dementia. *Health, Risk and Society* 2007; **9(4)**: 389–486.

14. Banerjee S, Willis R, Matthews D, *et al*. Improving the quality of care for mild to moderate dementia: an evaluation of the Croydon Memory Service Model. *International Journal of Geriatric Psychiatry* 2007; **22(8)**: 782–8.

15. Folstein MF, Folstein SE, McHugh PR. 'Mini-Mental State': a practical method for grading the cognitive state of patients for the clinician. *Journal of Psychiatry* 1975; **12(3)**: 189–98.

16. Brodaty H, Pond D, Kemp NM, *et al*. The GPCOG: a new screening test for dementia diagnosed for general practice. *Journal of the American Geriatrics Society* 2002; **50(3)**: 530–4.

17. Brooke P, Bullock R. Validation of a 6-item cognitive impairment test with a view to primary care usage. *International Journal of Geriatric Psychiatry* 1999; **14(11)**: 936–40.

18. Shulman KI, Shedletsky R, Silver I. The challenge of time: clock drawing and cognitive function in the elderly. *International Journal of Geriatric Psychiatry* 1986; **1(2)**: 135–40.

19. Milne A, Culverwell R, Guss J, *et al*. Screening for dementia in primary care: a review of the use, efficacy and quality of measures. *International Psychogeriatrics* 2008; **20(5)**: 911–26.

20. Alzheimer's Society. *Assessing Cognition in Older People: a practical toolkit for health professionals.* London: Alzheimer's Society, 2013, www.alzheimers.org.uk/site/scripts/documents_info. php?documentID=2159.

21. Bamford C, Lamont S, Eccles M, *et al.* Disclosing a diagnosis of dementia: a systematic review. *International Journal of Geriatric Psychiatry* 2004; **19(2)**: 151–69.

22. Iliffe S, Robinson AL, Brayne C, *et al.* Primary care and dementia: 1. diagnosis, screening and disclosure. *International Journal of Geriatric Psychiatry* 2009; **24(9)**: 895–901.

23. Moniz-Cook E, Manthorpe J. Personalising psychosocial interventions to individual needs and context. In: E Moniz-Cook, J Manthorpe (eds). *Early Psychosocial Intervention in Dementia: evidence-based practice psychosocial interventions in early dementia.* London: Jessica Kingsley Publishers; 2009, pp. 1–11.

24. National Council for Palliative Care. *Exploring Palliative Care for People with Dementia. A discussion document.* London: NCPC, 2006.

25. Hughes J C, Robinson L. General practice perspectives: co-ordinating end-of-life care. In: J C Hughes (ed.). *Palliative Care in Severe Dementia.* London: Quay Books, 2006, pp. 116–25.

26. Evans G E, Robinson L. The role of the family doctor in supportive care for people with dementia. In: JC Hughes, M Lloyd-Williams, GA Sachs (eds). *Supportive Care for the Person with Dementia.* Oxford: Oxford University Press, 2010, pp. 139–48.

27. Ahmedzai SH. The nature of palliation and its contribution to supportive care. In: SH Ahmedzai, M Muers (eds). *Supportive Care in Respiratory Disease.* Oxford: Oxford University Press, 2005, pp. 3–38.

28. National Institute for Health and Clinical Excellence. *Donepezil, Galantamine, Rivastigmine (Review) and Memantine for the Treatment of Alzheimer's Disease (Amended).* London: NICE, 2011.

29. O'Brien J, Robinson L, Fairbairn A. Proposed shared care protocol between primary and secondary care for the ongoing management of those on anti-dementia medication. *Journal of Primary Care Psychiatry* 2001; **7(3)**: 111–13.

30. Brodaty H, Green A, Koschera A. Meta-analysis of psychosocial interventions for caregivers of people with dementia. *Journal of the American Geriatrics Society* 2003; **51(5)**: 657–64.

31. Brodaty H, Thompson C, Fine M. Why caregivers of people with dementia and memory loss don't use services. *International Journal of Geriatric Psychiatry* 2005; **20(6)**: 537–46.

32. Fossey J, Ballard C, Juszczak E, *et al.* Effect of enhanced psychosocial care on antipsychotic use in nursing home residents with severe dementia: cluster randomised trial. *British Medical Journal* 2006; **332(7544)**: 756–61.

33. Schneider LS, Dagerman K, Insel PS. Efficacy and adverse effects of atypical antipsychotics for dementia: meta-analysis of randomized, placebo-controlled trials. *American Journal of Geriatric Psychiatry* 2006; **14(3)**: 191–210.

34. Ballard C, Margello LM, Theodoulou M, *et al.* A randomised, blinded, placebo-controlled trial in dementia patients continuing or stopping neuroleptics (the DART-AD trial). *PLoS Medicine* 2008; **5(4)**: e76.

35. Burns A, Iliffe S. Dementia. *British Medical Journal* 2009; **338**: 405–9.

36. Alzheimer's Society. *Optimising Treatment and Care for Behavioural and Psychological Symptoms of Dementia.* London: Alzheimer's Society, 2011, http://alzheimers.org.uk/site/scripts/documents_info.php?documentID=1657 [accessed July 2013].

37. Help the Aged, Peer Education Project Group. *Planning for Choice in End-of-Life Care: educational guide.* London: Help the Aged, 2006, www.hospice.co.uk/wp-content/uploads/2011/04/eolelderly.pdf [accessed July 2013].

38. Royal College of Physicians, National Council for Palliative Care, British Society of Rehabilitation Medicine, British Geriatrics Society, Alzheimer's Society, Royal College of Nursing, Royal College of Psychiatrists, Help the Aged, Royal College of General Practitioners. *Advance Care Planning.* Concise Guidance to Good Practice series, No 12. www.rcplondon.ac.uk/sites/default/files/documents/acp_web_final_21.01.09.pdf [accessed July 2013].

39. Henry C, Seymour J. *Advanced Care Planning: a guide for health and social care staff.* Leicester: End of Life Care Programme, 2009.

40. Exley C, Bamford C, Hughes J, *et al.* Advance Care Planning: an opportunity for patient centred care in dementia. *Dementia* 2009; **8(3)**: 419–24.

41. Department of Health. *The Mental Capacity Act 2005.* London: DH, 2005, http://webarchive.nationalarchives.gov.uk/+/www.dh.gov.uk/en/SocialCare/Deliveringadultsocialcare/MentalCapacity/MentalCapacityAct2005/index.htm [accessed July 2013].

42. Gold Standards Framework. *Prognostic Indicator Guidance to Aid Identification of Adult Patients with Advanced Disease, in the Last Months/Year of Life, Who Are in Need of Supportive and Palliative Care.* Shrewsbury: GSF, 2006, www.qrp.pops.net/iha_wg/d_coping_with_end_of_life/prognostic_indicators_guidance_paper.pdf [accessed July 2013].

43. Froggatt K, Vaughan S, Bernard C, *et al.* Advance care planning in care homes for older people: an English perspective. *Palliative Medicine* 2009; **23(4)**: 332–8.

44. Department of Health. *End of Life Care Strategy: promoting high quality care for all adults at the end of life.* London: DH, 2008.

45. Sampson E, Robinson AL. End of life care in dementia: building bridges for effective multidisciplinary care. *Dementia* 2009; **8(3)**: 331–4.

46. Robinson AL, Sampson EL. End of life care in dementia: research needed urgently to determine the acceptability and effectiveness of innovative approaches. *Dementia* 2009; **8(3)**: 418–19.

HIV and other blood-borne viruses

Surinder Singh and Paul Shire

The aim of this chapter is to outline the epidemiological and clinical aspects of the common blood-borne viral infections and in particular how this relates to patients in primary care. This chapter is divided into two main parts, first covering HIV infection and second the common types of viral hepatitis (A, B and C).

Key learning points

- HIV infection and other blood-borne viral infections such as hepatitis B and C can be carried for long periods before a person becomes unwell. During this time the infection can be transmitted to other individuals, including from mother to child *in utero*. People from disadvantaged backgrounds are invariably affected the most – black Africans, gay men, young people of both sexes, drug users and prisoners are some of the most vulnerable groups in the UK.

- It is now widely accepted in areas of high prevalence – where the prevalence of HIV is equal to or greater than 2:1000 – that it is appropriate to offer HIV testing for new registrants in general practice and all hospital admissions. There are compelling arguments for doing this; it is important to identify patients as early as possible in order to offer monitoring and treatment as necessary, and it makes economic sense (see first half of this chapter).

- Prevention is still a key message – and one that is easily forgotten. This means reinforcing messages about reducing risk and ensuring that co-infections are identified early.

- With regard to hepatitis, progression to cirrhosis can be reduced by effectively managing risk factors such as alcohol intake, obesity and preventing co-infection with HIV. Vaccination for hepatitis A and B should be offered to those at risk and to close contacts, using a rapid induction programme if necessary.

Overview of HIV infection and AIDS

Area of competence: primary care management. The most recent figures state that by the end of 2011 almost 96,000 people live with HIV infection in the UK[1,2] and while this appears to be a modest figure compared with other countries it is still significant. In 2011, 6280 new diagnoses of HIV were made in the UK. Overall, despite these figures, one might be forgiven for regarding the HIV issue as less important on account of major developments in antiretroviral therapies, resulting in a much better outlook for those with HIV infection.[3]

The at-risk groups described many years ago are really no different today. However, there is a more appropriate emphasis on risk behaviour. It is obvious that disadvantaged groups suffer most (see Box 8.1), for example people from migrant communities (black African and black Caribbean), men who have sex with men (MSM), prisoners or ex-prisoners and the young.[1,2] It is still the case that the highest number of new HIV diagnoses are reported in London, UK.

The undiagnosed group and the problem of late diagnosis

Area of competence: a comprehensive approach. There are approximately 22,600 individuals with HIV infection in the UK who have yet to be identified (24% of the total).[1] This is known through the anonymous unlinked HIV testing programme[1,4] and involves the collection of anonymous blood from individuals attending a range of sentinel clinics throughout the UK. In essence this programme provides critical public health information about how widespread HIV has become.

One highly perturbing feature of these statistics is that a good proportion of people who are newly diagnosed with HIV have advanced disease (see next section). Thus in 2009 over half of adults (3450/6630) aged over 15 years were diagnosed late (that is, they had a CD4 count below 350/per cubic mm within three months of diagnosis). Quite simply this means that it is too late for interventions such as antiretroviral therapy to work effectively.[5] This is why relatively recent guidance on HIV testing in the UK has emphasised the need to enhance testing, both in primary and secondary care (see next section). A key aim of this recent guidance is to reduce barriers to HIV testing and enhance the overall care of people with HIV by ensuring that a diagnosis is made earlier and that monitoring and treatment can begin in a timely manner.[6]

New testing policies

Area of competence: primary care management. Some commentators say that the UK's public health failure to diagnose almost a third of those with HIV infection and AIDS is appalling.[7,8] It is now accepted that in areas where the prevalence of HIV is 2:1000 this is a good enough reason to promote more widespread testing. Essentially this means that all medical admissions to hospital ought to be offered a test and also new patient registrations in general practice should be offered likewise.[9-11]

> ## Box 8.1 **Epidemiology of HIV in the UK (2008–11)**
>
> - In 2011 there were 6280 newly diagnosed with HIV in the UK – a 21% reduction from the peak in new diagnoses in 2005.[1]
>
> - 24% of people with HIV in the UK do not know they have HIV infection.[1]
>
> - New diagnoses among MSM have been increasing since 2007 with 3010 reports in 2011, representing an all-time high. There are both direct and indirect measures of incidence that the rate of HIV transmission in this population remains high.[1]
>
> - Over half of the 2900 heterosexual men and women diagnosed in 2011 probably acquired their HIV infection in the UK, compared with 27% in 2002.[1]
>
> - The number of new diagnoses among those infected heterosexually within the UK has remained steady (1100 per year since 2008). The number of new diagnoses among heterosexuals infected abroad continues to fall, from 3040 in 2008 to 2200 in 2010. This is largely due to a decrease in diagnoses among persons from sub-Saharan Africa. The latest HIV figures confirm that less than 1% of infants born to women diagnosed with HIV infection prior to delivery acquired perinatal infection in 2010/11.[1]
>
> - In 2011 an estimated 2300 people who inject drugs (PWID) were living with HIV in the UK, of whom about a fifth were unaware of their infection. The overall prevalence among PWID in England, Wales and Northern Ireland remained low in 2011, at approximately 1.2%. This figure is no different from 2010, which indicates transmission, albeit at a low level.[1]
>
> - Men who inject drugs who reported male sexual partners had a four-fold higher risk of being HIV-infected compared with male PWID who reported only sex with women.[1]
>
> - In England (2009 figures), the diagnosed prevalence of HIV was 3.7% among black Africans, nearly ten times higher than among black Caribbeans (0.4%) and over 40 times that among the white population (0.09).[12]
>
> - The black Caribbean community is disproportionately affected by bacterial sexually transmitted infections (STIs) and especially gonorrhoea. In 2007 this group accounted for over a quarter (26%) of heterosexually acquired gonorrhoea diagnosed in a sample of genitourinary medicine clinics in England and Wales.[12]

Such is the weight of evidence for this public health strategy that pilot schemes have taken place with the appropriate evaluations. Last but not least there is also a highly significant economic reason why late diagnosis is so 'costly', to the individual, family and society[13,14] – quite simply the earlier the diagnosis, the better the care that can be offered and provided, and the more effective it is.

Prevention of HIV

Area of competence: person-centred care. It is easy to forget the more traditional messages about safe sex and protecting oneself against HIV. However, the rise in sexually transmitted infections in the UK means that these messages are, to some extent, being unheeded (Box 8.2). Taking fewer risks, wearing condoms on every occasion, ensuring that people have regular checks and reporting symptoms early are some of the strategies being promoted by HIV/AIDS voluntary agencies. For those patients who are hepatitis B antibody positive other preventive measure may mean encouraging your partner to be vaccinated and again ensuring that risk-taking during sexual intercourse is minimised.

Box 8.2 Dispelling 'sexual health' myths [13]

Make sure you use reputable information. The following are urban myths surrounding HIV:

- HIV is only transmitted if you or your partner has an orgasm
- if you're the insertive partner then you can't become positive from the person being penetrated
- withdrawing from your partner before ejaculation prevents transmission.

People infected through injecting drug use make up about 2% of those with HIV/AIDS but prevention is still important.[1] Advice about alcohol, the encouragement to avoid injecting all street drugs and the use of clean needles are key parts of the prevention message. Importantly if injecting continues then clean equipment and no sharing are mandatory if further infection is to be avoided. It is recommended strongly that patients have hepatitis A and B vaccinations (see next section). Dual infections (hepatitis and HIV) are doubly difficult to treat and manage, with an increased level of morbidity for patients who are so affected.

The inner city

Area of competence: community orientation. The terms 'inner city' and 'disadvantage' seem to be inextricably linked.[1,15,16]

A constellation of factors such as high rates of migrants, poor housing, highly mobile populations, the homeless and people experiencing mental health symptoms make this a challenging place to work.[17,18] Case scenario 1 is an example of a patient with a new diagnosis (see below).

There is often a higher prevalence of people from prison – and it is known that prisoners have a higher rate of HIV infection and hepatitis than an average population.[15]

It is in such contexts where the new policy on testing will be most useful.[19] The overwhelmingly positive results of the rapidly implemented antenatal testing strategy in the mid-1990s means that widespread testing is possible and is effective.

Case scenario 1

DF was a 22-year-old Caucasian man with a nasty flu-like illness and for which he consulted the GP twice over ten days. He had had a sore throat, fever and mild rash, as well as a runny nose and general aches and pains. Although he was getting better by the second visit DF's major worry was that this might be related to recent travel but also to his 'homosexuality'. He admitted he had put himself at risk during the holiday, having had unprotected penetrative sex several times with different men.

In the surgery DF was 'poorly', with cough and rhinorrhoea, and he had a low-grade fever (temperature 38 degrees). He appeared anxious and restless – clearly worried about his health. He had not had any other symptoms but his main worry was that this was the onset of HIV infection.

An HIV test was requested but the earliest this could be done was the following morning. The doctor in the surgery called a specialist for advice and it was agreed that the patient be urgently reviewed in the HIV clinic the following afternoon. DF was diagnosed with HIV infection and this was the seroconversion illness.

It transpired that the man had lived with his parents in a small market town until the age of 15 years when he decided to 'come out'. This news was greeted with utter shock and complete rejection by his parents, and he went to live with a distant relative in London. He had tried to continue with further education and this was initially impossible to do, so he went travelling. It was at this point that he acquired HIV infection.

Making a diagnosis

How does one go about making a diagnosis of HIV infection? Quite simply this is about being aware of the condition and its many facets including AIDS-defining illnesses such as *Pneumocystis carinii* pneumonia (now re-named *Pneumocystis jiroveci*) and Kaposi's sarcoma. It is also important to be confident when talking about intimate subjects such as sex, lifestyle, sexual partners and practices, and past history, including STIs.

Specific communication strategies can help in thinking about the types of question to ask and tips can be found in both MEDFASH books.[18,20] Obviously the next thing to do is go ahead with the test, which is usually a blood test. Note in some places point-of-care testing is now becoming more available and for some purposes is a very useful tool.[21] This change in thinking around HIV infection means that testing becomes more 'normal' and that there is more of it in primary care. Importantly some of the features of patients that may alert you to the possibility of HIV infection include:

- having engaged in at-risk activity (MSM)

- having had an indicator disease (shingles, Bell's palsy, unusual infections)

- recent history of flu-like illness followed by physical deterioration

- unusual presentation of illnesses.

After the test

Area of competence: a comprehensive approach. It is beyond the scope of this chapter to discuss in detail the treatments for HIV and AIDS. This is adequately outlined in other texts.[22,23]

If the patient is HIV positive it is important that a discussion takes place about what should happen next. Often patients need time and a period of quiet reflection but the aim is to ensure that the patient is seen by a specialist unit within two days (though two weeks is the maximum waiting time according to national guidelines).[12] There are instances where this should be sooner – and this can only take place following a discussion with both patient and specialist.

If the individual is HIV negative then it is possible to give the result by telephone. It is recommended that the result is given in person to certain groups – for example those who are vulnerable, whose command of English is limited or who are very young (16 years).[12]

Primary HIV infection [18,20]

It is genuinely difficult to diagnose acute primary HIV infection, especially within a primary care setting where non-specific viral illnesses are so common all year round. Some of the factors that may alert the clinician to thinking about HIV are risk activity, recent travel, severity of illness and signs such as rash and/or cervical lymphadenopathy. The obvious advantages of identifying infection at this stage is that it is early (i.e. before infection is transmitted unwittingly) but that treatment can be offered. In all such cases a timely telephone call to the relevant on-call specialist should facilitate the patient being seen acutely.[7]

An HIV negative result also merits discussion. Some reference to why the test was being done in the first place is appropriate but advice about remaining negative is important, especially if the test was taken because of risk exposure. Importantly the 'window period' needs to be covered – in other words that a further test ought to be done if the risk was within the last month or so.

It may be sensible to provide advice about post-exposure prophy-laxis in certain instances, for example individuals who are at high risk of repeat exposure to HIV.[24]

Overview of viral hepatitis

Area of competence: primary care management. The prevalence of viral hepatitis in the UK, most commonly hepatitis A, B or C, is increasing. Many individuals who carry these illnesses are undiagnosed, which pre-vents them from accessing curative treatments and can place uninfected individuals at risk of acquiring the infection.

The majority of carriers of hepatitis B and C are from disadvantaged groups, such as drug users and migrants. Primary care practitioners are in an ideal position to identify patients at risk, undertake testing, and provide ongoing support to patients with chronic viral hepatitis.

Hepatitis A

Hepatitis A is now a rare infection in the UK. It is usually contracted during travel to endemic areas; however, outbreaks can occur in hos-tels, care facilities and in MSM. It is normally spread by the faecal–oral route. Since the introduction of a hepatitis A vaccination in the mid-1990s, reported cases of hepatitis A have dropped significantly.

Hepatitis A is usually identified when testing for acute hepatitis or in travellers with non-specific illness. The rate of fulminant liver fail-ure with hepatitis A is less than 1%, although this risk is higher in older people, and those with chronic liver disease or who have co-infection.[25] Hepatitis A never causes chronic liver disease.

Hepatitis B

Around 350 million people worldwide have chronic hepatitis B infection.[26] Prevalence of chronic infection is particularly high in China and Southeast Asia, the Amazon basin, the Middle East and Eastern Europe.[26] In the UK 0.3% of individuals are thought to have chronic hepatitis B;[27] however, the rates may be much higher in migrant communities.

Hepatitis B is transmitted by contact with infected blood or bodily fluids, so the most common routes of transmission are through sexual contact, contaminated equipment in drug use, sharps injuries, body art and through vertical transmission from mother to baby.

The majority of people are asymptomatic during the acute illness, and less than 1% will develop fulminant hepatitis. In adults, only 5% of individuals will develop chronic infection; however, this develops in 90% of children infected at birth and 25–30% infected between the ages of 1–4.[28] Between 15–40% of patients with chronic hepatitis B develop decompensated liver disease.[29,30]

Hepatitis C

Around 200,000 people are thought to be infected with chronic hepatitis C in the UK, with over half undiagnosed.[31] Hepatitis C is transmitted by contact with infected blood, and in the UK this is primarily through injecting drug use. It is thought that up to 50% of injecting drug users may be infected with hepatitis C.[32-34] The rate of transmission during sexual intercourse is much lower than for hepatitis B or HIV, although recent data suggest that this is still an important route of transmission in MSM.[35]

The majority of people infected with hepatitis C are asymptomatic during the acute phase of the illness. This makes detection of hepatitis C difficult, and individuals can present with decompensated liver disease or hepatocellular carcinoma as the first indication of infection. Up to 85% of individuals affected will progress to having chronic infection, with around 20% going on to develop cirrhosis; however, this may take many years to develop.[32-34] The development of cirrhosis increases with duration of infection and is considerably accelerated by excessive alcohol consumption.

Identification and testing

Areas of competence: community orientation and person-centred care. The recent structural changes to the NHS have increased the role of GPs in commissioning health care. It will be vital to ensure that funding remains in place for public health campaigns, and for drug and sexual health services that are easily accessible by marginalised groups. Clinical Commissioning Groups (CCGs) should be well placed to understand the needs of the local community they serve. The National Institute for Health and Care Excellence published guidance in 2012 on the ways to promote and offer hepatitis B and C testing.[36]

A new patient consultation is an ideal opportunity to offer screening to high-risk groups, especially migrants and anyone who has ever injected drugs. *Ad hoc* testing should also be considered for the groups listed in Box 8.3. Posters and reading material highlighting risk factors can encourage patients to raise their concerns with doctors or nursing staff at the practice.

Box 8.3 Patient groups to whom testing for hepatitis (B and C) should be offered [28, 29]

- Anyone with unexplained abnormal liver function tests or unexplained jaundice.
- Anyone who has injected drugs in the past (including anabolic steroids) using shared equipment, even if it was just once or twice.
- Anyone who received a blood transfusion in the UK before 1991 (or blood products before 1986).
- Individuals if they have received medical or dental treatment in countries where infection control may be poor.
- Child of a mother with hepatitis.
- Regular sexual partner of someone with hepatitis B or C.
- Has had tattoos, body piercing, acupuncture or electrolysis where infection control may be poor.

In general practice, where the individual's history is often known, a brief pre-test discussion to undertake a risk assessment and explain the benefits of the test is appropriate. The Department of Health has published a very useful two-page reference guide for primary care that gives targeted advice on pre- and post-test discussions.[35] HIV testing can also be offered following these discussions.

Blood-borne virus testing has become a routine feature in drugs services in the UK and is offered in genitourinary medicine clinics; however, it is vital to ensure that this has been considered when seeing a patient who is a drug user in primary care for the first time.

Case scenario 2

In 2007, a 45-year-old woman (BD), presented to the GP with tiredness and difficulty sleeping. After a focused history and examination, routine blood tests were requested that revealed a marked rise in liver enzymes. After several attempts to contact BD, she made an appointment and talked about her ongoing abusive relationship, alcohol misuse, joint pains and longstanding psoriasis. She revealed that in the past she had 'dabbled in drugs' and once a doctor did tell her she was at risk of hepatitis C.

She agreed to be tested for hepatitis. Her liver function tests were still raised and hepatitis C antibody was confirmed; there was no co-infection. Unfortunately, despite several reminders and a home visit it was not possible to contact the patient again (even though she was still 'registered' at the practice).

One of the challenges of working in the inner city, where patient turnover is often 35–40% per year, is that follow-up can be extremely difficult. If she was to ever re-engage with us it would be appropriate to refer her to a liver specialist and to discuss minimising co-infection and mitigating her hepatitis by reducing alcohol intake. It would also be prudent to try to help BD regarding the domestic violence, which probably goes some way to explaining the past drug and alcohol abuse and previous hepatitis.

Prevention and harm reduction

Area of competence: person-centred care. Injecting drug use is the most significant risk factor for hepatitis C, and is also a significant risk factor for hepatitis B. Drug users engaged with specialist services, using substitution therapies as well as clean drug equipment, are at lower risk of transmission.

The UK currently runs a selective vaccination policy for hepatitis B.[36] Co-infection with hepatitis A, B, C or HIV results in more severe or progressive liver disease. Hepatitis A and B vaccination is offered to individuals at high risk for co-infection, including drug users, those with chronic liver or renal disease, confirmed viral hepatitis, prisoners, MSM and in certain occupational circumstances.[37] They are also offered to travellers visiting countries with high prevalence. The schedules for hepatitis B can be accelerated, especially if the person could move elsewhere, to improve completion rates.[37]

Advice should be offered about safer sex, condom use and not to share razors or toothbrushes. New or existing partners of individuals with hepatitis B and household contacts should be tested and offered vaccination.

In patients diagnosed with chronic hepatitis, it is important that modifiable factors that increase risk of progression to cirrhosis are regularly addressed within primary and secondary care. The rate of progression to end-stage liver disease can be reduced by minimising alcohol intake and ideally abstaining if possible. Patients who are obese should be given support to achieve a healthy body mass index (BMI).

Diagnosis and treatment

Area of competence: primary care management. The initial blood tests required for diagnosis are hepatitis B surface antigen (HBsAg) (not to be confused with its antibody HBsAb), and hepatitis C antibody. If a positive result is obtained, a confirmatory sample should be sent along with samples for viral load and hepatitis C genotype. If HBsAg is positive, it is good practice to request a test for the delta particle of hepatitis D.

Acute viral hepatitis usually requires supportive care only, but specialist input may be needed if a patient has severe symptoms or grossly deranged liver function tests. Chronic hepatitis B is diagnosed with the continued presence of HBsAg after six months. There are a number of other antigen and antibody tests that give an indication of the stage of infection and degree of infectivity.[38] On the rare occasion where acute hepatitis C is diagnosed (for example after a needle stick injury), it may be possible to treat this with pegylated interferon, thus avoiding a chronic infection.

Chronic hepatitis C is confirmed if a patient tests positive for hepatitis C antibody and there is ongoing presence of hepatitis C viral RNA in the blood. If a negative hepatitis C antibody test has been obtained, but the patient is concerned about a recent exposure, the test should be repeated after a minimum of three months. After infection with hepatitis C, the antibody test will remain positive for many years. If the PCR test for viral RNA is negative, the infection has cleared spontaneously. However, this does not afford any protection against later re-infection. It is important to ensure that patients understand this.

Chronic hepatitis B or C should be managed by a specialist in viral hepatitis – though arrangements to establish links with primary care are essential, especially if the disease is unstable or progressive (see case scenario 3, overleaf).

Post-exposure prophylaxis is available for hepatitis B and current guidance[39-41] is useful in this instance. Vertical transmission of hepatitis B can be reduced by 90% through the combination of hepatitis B immunoglobulin and hepatitis B vaccination given to the neonate.

A range of medications exists for treatment of hepatitis B, including interferon alfa and a number of nucleoside analogues. A full NICE guideline for chronic hepatitis B is expected in 2013. Treatments usually result in viral suppression rather than clearance, but it is generally recommended if there is advanced disease or high viral loads. Individuals with mild disease may be kept under surveillance.

Clearer guidelines exist for the treatment of hepatitis C.[42,43] Viral clearance rates in hepatitis C can be as high as 55–90%, depending on genotype. Genotypes 1 and 4 have lower sustained viral response (SVR) rates than genotypes 2 and 3. Treatment can also reduce progression to advanced stages of liver disease. The most common treatment for hepatitis C is the combination of pegylated interferon and ribavirin. Two protease inhibitors, telaprevir and boceprevir, have been evaluated by NICE and are now available in combination with the standard treatments for genotype 1 hepatitis C infection.[44,45] There are numerous agents in stage 3 clinical trials, and there is considerable hope for long-term improvements in clearance rates, with less toxic and shorter treatment regimes.

It is important to know the common side effects of antiviral treatments. Pegylated interferon can cause a persistent influenza-like illness, anaemia, thrombocytopenia, thyroid disorders and mood disturbances. Ribavirin can cause haemolytic anaemia and is teratogenic. Effective contraception is vital while on these treatments and for six months afterwards.

Clinical nurse specialists play a crucial role in supporting patients with hepatitis, especially those on antiviral therapies. Their role also encompasses harm reduction, advice on alcohol and drug services, and education. Importantly it is the clinical nurse specialists who often liaise with primary care.

Long-term complications

....

Case scenario 3

A 40-year-old African man (BS), married with two young children, presented in 2008 with a two-year history of intermittent epigastric pain and recent melaena. He had been registered since 2004, but rarely consulted. He drank 1–2 bottles of wine a week, but had previously drunk more. He had no prior history of jaundice, hepatitis or receipt of a blood transfusion. Abdominal tribal markings and hepatomegaly were noted.

He was found to have a profound pancytopenia, and he had markedly raised liver function tests. He was admitted into hospital and underwent an upper GI endoscopy, ultrasound and CT scanning. His final diagnoses included oesophageal varices, liver cirrhosis secondary to hepatitis B infection and a single large hepatocellular carcinoma, not amenable to surgery.

He has undergone a number of cycles of transarterial chemoembolisation (TACE), which delivers chemotherapeutic agents via the hepatic artery. Sorafenib has been used, but it has been limited by the development of hand and foot skin reactions. His treatment is ongoing but palliative in nature; the prognosis is poor.

BS originally presented with complications of advanced liver disease and he is likely to have carried hepatitis B infection for many years. If it had been identified earlier, the risk of advanced liver disease could have been reduced, and surgical removal of the tumour may have been possible. Importantly, messages about alcohol intake and vaccination of household contacts are easily forgotten, especially in the acute circumstances.

Area of competence: community orientation. Patients with chronic hepatitis need long-term surveillance to detect signs of cirrhosis as the rate of progression is usually slow. Transplantation is an option in decompensated liver failure. Individuals with cirrhosis should have six-monthly ultrasound and alfafetoprotein levels to screen for the development of hepatocellular carcinoma, although the evidence to confirm this significantly lengthens life expectancy or achieves cost savings is lacking.[46]

Between 1–4% of individuals with cirrhosis develop hepatocellular carcinoma per year.[46] If identified early, hepatocellular carcinoma can be treated by liver resection or transplantation; however, most patients present with symptoms of advanced hepatocellular carcinoma or decompensated liver disease, and treatment is usually palliative only.

Useful resources

- MEDFASH, Medical Foundation for AIDS & Sexual Health
  c/o BMA House, Tavistock Square, London WCIH 9JP
  Website: www.medfash.org.uk

- Terrence Higgins Trust
  314–320 Gray's Inn Road, London WC1X 8DP
  Phone: 0845 122 1200 | Website: www.tht.org.uk

- British HIV Association (BHIVA)
  BHIVA Secretariat, 1 Mountview Court, 310 Friern Barnet Lane, London N20 0LD
  Website: www.bhiva.org

- Public Health England
  Wellington House, 133–155 Waterloo Road, London SE1 8UG
  Website: www.gov.uk/government/organisations/public-health-england/

- British Liver Trust
  2 Southampton Road, Ringwood, Hampshire BH24 1HY
  Website: www.britishlivertrust.org.uk

- Hepatitis Advisory Service
  41 Norval Road, North Wembley, Middlesex HA0 3TD
  Phone: 0800 206 1899 | Website: www.hepbpositive.org.uk

- National AIDS Trust (NAT)
  New City Cloisters, 196 Old Street, London EC1V 9FR
  Phone: 44 020 7814 6767 | Website: www.nat.org.uk

References

1. Health Protection Agency. *HIV in the United Kingdom: 2012 report*. London: Health Protection Services, 2012, www.hpa.org.uk/webc/HPAwebFile/HPAweb_C/1317137200016 [accessed July 2013].

2. Health Protection Agency. *Time to Test for HIV: expanded healthcare and community HIV-testing in England*. London: HPA, www.hpa.org.uk/webc/HPAwebFile/HPAweb_C/1287145497243 [accessed July 2013].

3. Antiretroviral Therapy Cohort Collaboration. Life expectancy of individuals on combination antiretroviral therapy in high-income countries: a collaborative analysis of 14 cohort studies. *Lancet* 2008; **372(9635)**: 293–9.

4. Information about the anonymous unlinked programme for HIV testing, www.hpa.org.uk/web/HPAweb&Page&HPAwebAutoListName/Page/1201094588821 [accessed July 2013].

5. Health Protection Agency. *HIV in the United Kingdom: 2010 report*. London: HPA, 2010, www.hpa.org.uk/webc/HPAwebFile/HPAweb_C/1287145367237 [accessed July 2013].

6. National Institute for Health and Clinical Excellence. *Increasing the Uptake of HIV Testing among Black Africans in England* (Public Health Guidance 33). London: NICE, 2011, www.nice.org.uk/guidance/PH33 [accessed August 2013].

7. Hamill M, Burgoine K, Farrell F, *et al*. Time to move towards opt-out testing for HIV in the UK. *British Medical Journal* 2007; **334(7608)**: 1352–4

8. The UK's appalling failure to tackle HIV [editorial]. *Lancet* 209; **373(9678)**: 1820.

9. Bryce G. HIV testing in primary care [editorial]. *British Medical Journal* 2009; **338**: b1085, http://dx.doi.org/10.1136/bmj.b1085 [accessed August 2013].

10. Public Health England. *HIV Epidemiology in London: 2011 data*. London: PHE, 2013, www.hpa.org.uk/webc/HPAwebFile/HPAweb_C/1317138999825 [accessed July 2013].

11. Health Protection Agency. *Sexually Transmitted Infections in Black African and Black Caribbean Communities in the UK: 2008 report*. London: HPA, www.hpa.org.uk/webc/HPAwebFile/HPAweb_C/1225441603957 [accessed July 2013].

12. British HIV Association, British Association of Sexual Health and HIV, British Infection Society. *UK National Guidelines for HIV Testing 2008*. London: BHIVA, www.bashh.org/documents/1838.pdf [accessed July 2013].

13. Terrence Higgins Trust, information resources (2012), www.tht.org.uk/sexual-health/HIV-STIs/sex-and-risk/reduce-your-risk [accessed 20.5.2013]

14. National Institute for Health and Clinical Excellence. *Increasing the Uptake of HIV Testing among Men Who Have Sex with Men* (Public Health Guidance 34). London: NICE, 2011, www.nice.org.uk/guidance/PH34 [accessed July 2013].

15. National AIDS Trust, Terrence Higgins Trust. *Poverty and HIV 2006–2009*. London: NAT, 2010, www.nat.org.uk/media/Files/Publications/Sep-2010-Poverty-and-HIV-2006-2009.pdf [accessed July 2013].

16. Singh S. General practice and patient Y. *Journal of the Royal Society of Medicine* 1999; **92 (2)**: 94.

17. HIV in the United Kingdom (2012 figures), www.hpa.org.uk/webc/HPAwebFile/HPAweb_C/1317137200234 [accessed July 2013].

18. Madge S, Matthews P, Singh S, *et al*. *HIV in Primary Care* (2nd edn). London: MEDFASH, 2011, www.medfash.org.uk/uploads/files/p17abjng1g9t9193h1rsl75uuk53.pdf [accessed July 2013].

19. National AIDS Trust. *HIV Testing Action Plan to Reduce Late HIV Diagnosis in the UK* (2nd edn). London: NAT, 2012, www.nat.org.uk/media/Files/Policy/2012/May-2012-Testing-Action-Plan.pdf [accessed July 2013].

20. Baggaley R. *HIV for Non-HIV Specialists: diagnosing the undiagnosed*. London: MEDFASH, 2008, www.medfash.org.uk/uploads/files/p17am0h8v510dr1f941ebg1sicgpr.pdf [accessed July 2013].

21. National AIDS Trust. Types of HIV test (policy briefing), 2011. www.nat.org.uk/media/Files/Publications/Oct-2011-Types-of-HIV-test.pdf [accessed July 2013].

22. Gazzard B G on behalf of the BHIVA Treatment Guidelines Writing Group. British HIV Association guidelines for the treatment of HIV-1-infected adults with antiretroviral therapy 2008. *HIV Medicine* 2008; **9**: 563–608, www.bhiva.org/documents/Guidelines/Treatment%20Guidelines/Current/TreatmentGuidelines2008.pdf [accessed July 2013].

23. Addendum to BHIVA treatment guidelines (2009), www.bhiva.org/AddendumtoTreatmentGuidelines.aspx [accessed July 2013].

24. Fisher M, Benn P, Evans B, *et al*. UK guideline for the use of post-exposure prophylaxis for HIV following sexual exposure. *International Journal of STD & AIDS* 2006; **17 (2)**: 81–92, www.bashh.org/documents/58/58.pdf [accessed July 2013].

25. Crowcroft N S, Walsh B, Davison K L, *et al*. on behalf of the PHLS Advisory Committee. Guidelines for the control of hepatitis A virus infection. *Communicable Disease and Public Health* 2001; **4 (3)**: 213–17, www.hpa.org.uk/cdph/issues/CDPHvol4/No3/HepAguidelines0901.pdf [accessed July 2013].

26. World Health Organization. Fact sheet No. 204, Hepatitis B (2013), www.who.int/mediacentre/factsheets/fs204/en/ [accessed July 2013].

27. Health Protection Agency. General information on hepatitis B (2009), www.hpa.org.uk/Topics/InfectiousDiseases/InfectionsAZ/HepatitisB/GeneralInformationHepatitisB/hepbGeneralInfo/ [accessed July 2013].

28. English P. Should universal hepatitis B immunisation be introduced in the UK? *Archives of Disease in Childhood* 2006; **91 (14)**: 286–9.

29. Liaw Y F, Tai D I, Chu C M, *et al*. The development of cirrhosis in patients with chronic type B hepatitis: a prospective study. *Hepatology* 1988; **8 (3)**: 493–6.

30. Aggarwal R, Ranjan P. Preventing and treating hepatitis B infection. *British Medical Journal* 2004; **329 (7474)**: 1080–6.

31. Department of Health. *Hepatitis C: essential information for professionals and guidance on testing*. London: DH, 2004, www.nhs.uk/Livewell/hepatitisc/Documents/Information-for-professionals-19.05.061for-web-15600.pdf [accessed July 2013].

32. Health Protection Agency. *Hepatitis C in the UK: 2011 report*. London: HPA, www.hpa.org.uk/web/HPAwebFile/HPAweb_C/1309969906418 [accessed July 2013].

33. Nash KL, Bentley I, Hirschfield GM. Managing hepatitis C virus infection. *British Medical Journal* 2009; **338**: 37–42.

34. Department of Health. *Hepatitis C Action Plan for England*. London: DH, 2004, http://webarchive.nationalarchives.gov.uk/+/www.dh.gov.uk/en/Publicationsandstatistics/Publications/Publicationspolicyandguidance/DH_4084521 [accessed July 2013].

35. Health Protection Agency. *Hepatitis C in London: annual review (2011 data)*. London: HPA, 2012, www.hpa.org.uk/webc/HPAwebFile/HPAweb_C/1317135974202 [accessed July 2013].

36. National Institute for Health and Clinical Excellence. *Hepatitis B and C: ways to promote and offer testing to people at increased risk of infection* (Public Health Guidance 43). London: NICE, 2012, www.nice.org.uk/PH43 [accessed July 2013].

37. Department of Health. Hepatitis C: quick reference guide for primary care (2009), www.nhs.uk/Livewell/hepatitisc/Documents/hep_c_quick_ref_guide_for_primary_care.pdf [accessed July 2013].

38. Salisbury D, Ramsay M, Noakes K (eds). *Immunisation against Infectious Disease* ('the Green Book') (3rd edn). London: HMSO, 2006.

39. Coffey E, Young D. *Guidance for Hepatitis A and B Vaccination of Drug Users in Primary Care and Criteria for Audit*. London: RCGP, 2005, www.smmgp.org.uk/download/guidance/guidance014.pdf [accessed July 2013].

40. GP notebook. Hepatitis B serology, www.gpnotebook.co.uk/simplepage.cfm?ID=-80412651 [accessed July 2013].

41. PHLS Subcommittee. Exposure to hepatitis B virus: guidance on post-exposure prophylaxis. *Communicable Disease Report CDR Review* 1992; **2(9)**: R97–101. www.hpa.org.uk/cdr/archives/CDRreview/1992/cdrr0992.pdf [accessed July 2013].

42. Booth JCL, O'Grady J, Neuberger J. *Clinical Guidelines on the Management of Hepatitis C*. London: BSG, 2001, www.bsg.org.uk/images/stories/docs/clinical/guidelines/liver/clinguidehepc.pdf [accessed July 2013].

43. Scottish Intercollegiate Guidelines Network. *Management of Hepatitis C*. Edinburgh: SIGN, 2006, www.sign.ac.uk/pdf/sign92.pdf [accessed July 2013].

44. National Institute for Health and Clinical Excellence. *Telaprevir for the Treatment of Genotype 1 Chronic Hepatitis C* (Technology Appraisal 252). London: NICE, 2012, http://guidance.nice.org.uk/TA252 [accessed July 2013].

45. National Institute for Health and Clinical Excellence. *Boceprevir for the Treatment of Genotype 1 Chronic Hepatitis C* (Technology Appraisal 253). London: NICE, 2012, http://guidance.nice.org.uk/TA253 [accessed July 2013].

46. Ryder SD. Guidelines for the diagnosis and treatment of hepatocellular carcinoma (HCC) in adults. *Gut* 2003; **52 (Suppl 3)**: iii1–8, www.bsg.org.uk/pdf_word_docs/hcc.pdf [accessed July 2013].

9 Caring for patients with intellectual disabilities

Graham Martin

Aim

The aim of this chapter is to highlight inequalities in care received by those with an intellectual disability. The chapter gives an overview of the prevalence and clinical presentation of intellectual disability in primary care, subsequent investigation and the key areas of primary care management of this and related conditions. These areas include consent, holistic care and treatment options, whereby inequalities may be reduced.

Key learning points

- There is extensive evidence that many people with intellectual disabilities (PWID) are at a disadvantage because of access, communication, sensory and comprehension issues.

- In addition to the underlying cause of the learning disability, PWID are likely to have associated medical conditions, which may not be obvious (diagnostic overshadowing).

- Access, attitude and continuity issues may aggravate any health shortfall in their care.

- This shortfall (health inequality) may be reduced by allocating extra time, engaging more fully, and ensuring the patient's agenda is addressed.

- A planned, comprehensive annual health check in protected time may further reduce any inequality gap.

Introduction

No two patients are identical and some of the difference is due to biological variation and/or patient choice. Where there is a 'knock on' effect consequent upon biological variation, which merges into disability and disease conditions, then health inequality may merge into health inequity if inappropriate management leads to unjust and unfair treatment. Julian Tudor Hart observed that communities most in need of good care were least likely to get it.[1] The population of those with intellectual disabilities, who have limited cognitive ability, impaired ability to socially function without some help from another person, and whose lifelong condition was present before age 18, probably form one such population, though they are scattered in an irregular distribution throughout the primary care system. Each GP should be caring for an average of about eight patients with clinically important intellectual disability and a further 2% of the practitioner's patients will have mild or borderline learning disability. The terms intellectual disability and learning disability are for most purposes interchangeable in the UK.

In the general population, from a chronological point of view, mobility problems and dementia are more common at the upper end of the chronological spectrum and appropriate services exist to meet these needs, targeted towards the upper end of the age range. In this situation there is health inequality but an equitable solution is usually found for the actual health need of such populations.

By contrast, with decreasing intelligence quotient in a population there appears to be increasing disadvantage to the individual. Increasing severity of learning disabilities is associated with negative factors that cascade together to make health inequity (unnecessary, unjust and unfair health inequality) more and more likely. In particular, because of their increasing lack of autonomy and dependence on carers, with increasing severity of intellectual disability comes increasing inability to navigate the primary care system effectively without support. In addition to difficulties with literacy, inability to cope with going online may further widen the health inequality gap when lack of competency in information technology, or even ownership of a computer, is factored in.

The role of supporting carers for several aspects of social functioning in the community is pivotal. But equally, in clinical matters, identical treatment of patients is not possible or desirable, due to biopsychosocial diversity. Appropriate assessment of an individual's actual clinical and related needs must be made before a definitive clinical management plan can be agreed with patient and carer.

The health inequalities that matter here, and potentially can be changed, are 'unjust or unfair differences in health determinants or outcomes within or between defined populations'.[2]

Health inequalities can be tackled at an individual level if and when patients present with clinical problems. There is evidence however of additional unaddressed clinical needs, and twice the number of clinical needs may be identified by a structured annual health check compared with standard GP care.[3,4] So, in the group, as opposed to the individual situation, a practice learning disability population register and the offer of annual health checks should help to reduce the inequality gap for these patients.[5]

The factors associated with health inequality in people with learning disabilities are complex and interrelated, and include some more patient-oriented, and some more clinician-oriented, features. These features, some of which may be modified, may either widen or narrow the inequality/inequity gap. For the purposes of discussion, four areas centred on the patient, and four areas more approached from clinician/carer perspective, are listed below. These eight possible areas of health inequalities are considered, then the same areas are approached from the perspective of how they may be managed, to reduce the health inequalities issues.

Patient-centred issues

- Limited cognitive ability (low IQ).
- Sensory and communication difficulties.
- Features of the underlying causative condition.
- Frequently associated medical conditions.

Support-centred issues

- Consent and choice.
- Care arrangements (contextual issues).
- Access, attitude and continuity issues in primary care.
- Diagnostic overshadowing.

Consideration of intellectual disability issues in primary care

Limited cognitive ability

The principal reason why PWID are disadvantaged centres around their increasing inability to coherently inform clinicians why they may be distressed, and for their inability to understand proposed treatments. We ourselves may have difficulty describing the nature of abdominal pains or symptoms such as nausea; this is often much harder for PWID who may have a limited or no vocabulary. Abdominal discomfort is probably as common a symptom in PWID as in the general community, but PWID are less likely to have the skills to obtain, for example, over-the-counter (OTC) medications or to understand how to use them, particularly in a 'p.r.n.' situation. With those with severe and profound intellectual disabilities, they may respond atypically to distress or discomfort as they do not have the usual language with which to express their feelings.

Sensory and communication difficulties

PWID frequently have impairment of their sensory functions, particularly hearing and sight. They are less likely to be able to use glasses and hearing aids, so, in conjunction with limited cognitive ability, are less likely to be able to read instructions or understand explanatory diagrams. People with Down's syndrome may be difficult to understand due to problems in phonation due to variations in tongue and mouth structure, and they may also have impaired hearing.

Syndrome-specific and other features of underlying conditions

Some conditions are known to have commonly associated problems. For example, patients with Down's syndrome could well have hypothyroidism, congenital heart disease, hearing difficulties or dementia; coeliac disease and blood disorders may also occur. People with fragile X syndrome may well have social anxiety. A patient with cerebral palsy is quite likely to have mobility problems and epilepsy.

Associated common medical conditions

Many people with learning disability have raised body mass index (BMI) and fail to take adequate exercise, although others, usually with mild learning disabilities, should be able to diet appropriately, exercise and keep fit. Patients with ambulation difficulties may develop osteoporosis earlier than expected. Patients taking some anticonvulsants may also be more prone to osteoporosis.

Reflux, constipation and H. pylori infections are found more commonly than one would expect, particularly in PWID who have been in institutional care, or who are in residential care homes.

Gastric carcinoma is also found more commonly than expected. Some medical conditions occur equally frequently in the non-disabled population, but overall medical conditions are 2.5 times as common in those with learning disabilities; this does not include the condition of learning disability itself, but does include central nervous system (CNS) conditions, particularly epilepsy, gastrointestinal disorders[6] and diabetes.

Support-centred issues

Consent and 'choice'

Consideration of the matter of consent and choice, while not directly a cause of inequality, may nevertheless lead to difficulties. Where urgent treatment is needed, delay may occur if it is felt necessary to obtain consent involving a third party, for example delay to obtain consent before performing a life-saving procedure, such as operating to remove a gangrenous appendix.

A profoundly disabled patient, who is unable to understand what is being done or why it is necessary, doesn't willingly choose to cooperate. For example, not cooperating with normal hygienic procedures such as teeth brushing could be regarded as failing to consent. Consider a patient with profound learning disabilities who sometimes tries to avoid having his or her regular teeth brushing. The failure to see that teeth and gums are brushed regularly might be reckoned by care staff to be because the patient has 'chosen' not to have it done. This could lead to gingivitis and eventual dental extraction/clearance rather than the tedious but necessary hard work of conservation, involving minimum constraint necessary. There needs to be a carefully struck balance in interventions to counter the charges of unnecessary actions, on the one hand, and neglect, on the other.

Adults are assumed to be autonomous, that is, able to make rational decisions and consequently to consent to investigations or treatments, but this is not always so for PWID. PWID, particularly with severe or profound intellectual disability, may be unable to understand information relevant to a decision, to retain that information to weigh it and to communicate their decision by reason of an impairment or disturbance of the functioning of the mind. Therefore, other people with a duty of care towards the patient, for example family or paid carers, as well as clinicians, should probably be involved in the decision-making process in the best interests of the patient, and such decisions should be recorded.

Care arrangements (contextual issues)

A significant proportion of PWID live in residential care homes; often staff have no clinical background although they should have basic training. The staff of day centres may be likewise not fully aware of the medical needs of their service users. Those PWID who live in supported tenancies, again a significant number, have only intermittent supervision, and may decide to seek medical help or advice when no supervising carer is directly available. Conversely they may delay seeking appropriate help when there is 'no one to ask'. Although carers present at consultations usually are able very helpfully to augment information from the PWID, they could occasionally bias the outcome of consultations if their own agenda differs from that of the PWID.

Attitude, availability, access, continuity of care

Of 1000 people with mental health problems and/or learning disabilities responding to a consultation questionnaire from the Disability Rights Commission in 2005, over half reported difficulties in trying to use the services provided by their doctor's surgery. These difficulties included the attitude of reception staff, some clinical staff neglecting physical health problems by focusing only on the person's psychiatric condition or learning disability, problems with inflexible appointment systems, and inaccessible information and communications.[7] Medical staff in some situations may treat PWID less thoroughly, thinking the person's quality of life is less than that of the non-disabled. Such non-clinical value judgements, which cannot be justified, deprive the PWID of a level of health to which they should expect to be entitled.

Diagnostic overshadowing

As indicated above, the immediate presenting features of a PWID and their underlying condition may distract the clinician from properly investigating presenting symptoms. For example, bizarre behaviour such as head banging could be put down to the patient's severe intellectual disabilities whereas in fact it is due to earache or toothache.

Management options: what can be done to reduce health inequalities?

Adapting to limited cognitive ability

Where a patient has a very low IQ, the history is often given indirectly via a carer. It should be corroborated much more carefully than usual, by reference to past history if available. Some patients may simply reply 'yes' to all questions, which is misleading; their actual comprehension needs checking by asking the same question in a different way. Near patient tests such as measuring for fever, urine dipsticks and, where appropriate, blood tests, etc. will be required more often than with patients who can give a complete and accurate history. Careful observation of the patient and his or her body language may help to indicate the reason for the problem; for example, a mute patient with profound learning disability with abdominal colic might lie curled up, be pale and seem preoccupied. Exceptionally, a few may attempt distraction from their pain by self-inflicted biting to fingers or hands.

Reducing sensory and communication difficulties

Checking the hearing and inspecting for impacted wax should be regular parts of assessment. Care in examination and syringing need to be exercised in patients with Down's syndrome where the external auditory meatus may be shorter than is usual. Using hearing aids, speaking slowly, clearly and simply to the patient, and giving adequate time for a response are helpful. Checking the answer by a further question may help to validate the answer given (see above). The services of a specialist speech and language therapist may be helpful either in assessment or in communication situations. Some PWID are able to communicate using Makaton or other signing methods. Some PWID may have a short attention span and may be easily distracted.

Advice sheets can be used, such as the ones available to download from the Easy Health website (www.easyhealth.org.uk). There are also books specially written and illustrated for PWID, such as the Royal College of Psychiatrists' 'Books beyond Words' series. Both are helpful in appropriate situations.

Recognising features of the underlying causative condition

A knowledge of associated features of syndromes and other underlying causative conditions may help in the monitoring and management of patients with intellectual disabilities. For example, a middle-aged patient with Down's syndrome who seems to have become less active and is often sleeping might need to have his or her thyroid function tests measured. However, the patient might also be starting to have dementia or depression; the dose of anticonvulsant might need to be changed.

Awareness of associated common medical conditions

Exercise may be prescribed for some PWID who are overweight and/or physically unfit, and who may not be motivated to exercise. Some patients with severe intellectual disabilities may benefit from specific postural advice and physiotherapy. BMI tends to be higher than in the general population and fluids may be increased, diet may be improved and exercise prescribed to reduce obesity and constipation, and to increase fitness.

Over 90% of patients with learning disabilities in long-term residential care test positive for H. pylori. Although some may not be able satisfactorily to perform a breath test, serum or stool tests may confirm H. pylori. Reflux and kyphoscoliosis are also more common in patients with cerebral palsy than in the general population. Tilting the head of the bed up by about 15 cm may reduce reflux.[8,9] Some may feel there is a case for triple therapy and possibly (long-term) proton pump inhibitors (PPIs), with or without a definitive diagnosis.

Consent

As indicated above, passive assent may not be assumed for a course of treatment, the risks and implications of which cannot be understood by the patient. Nevertheless the duty of care means that those involved in the ongoing care of a patient who cannot make his or her own decisions must make and implement clinical decisions in the best interests of the PWID after appropriate consultation and making a record of the reasons (see Chapter 7, p. 116).

Arrangements for care and place of residence

Because some PWID spend their day at day centres and evenings and nights at their residential care home, it may be difficult to arrange for them to attend surgeries at a time most convenient to the GP. However, mid-afternoon, when they are transferring between day centre and home may be a suitable time; transport may have been organised in any case and a carer may be accompanying the patient.

Home visits outside of normal working hours may be of value to see patients in their usual surroundings, particularly for patients who cannot walk and where time is needed to check their multiple co-morbidities. Some patients, for example those with fragile X, can become socially very anxious. Surgery waiting room times need to be kept to a minimum particularly for this patient group.

Improving access, attitude and continuity of care

People with learning disabilities may find it difficult to adapt to new carers and clinicians, so personal continuity of care is very important. Additionally, as deafness is very common, or can itself be a reason for the appointment, PWID would prefer the doctor or nurse to come out of their consulting rooms to invite them in, rather than to depend on an impersonal electronic screen and/or automated voice system. Before a visit to the doctor, a carer should write down any patient concerns and prepare the patient before examination or other procedure; it is particularly important that a trusted person explains to the PWID what is about to happen. Appendix A on p. 152 shows a pre-health check questionnaire for patients with learning disabilities.

Awareness of diagnostic overshadowing

While unusual behaviour could be due to the patient's learning disabilities, any new or variant behaviour should never be explained as simply due to the learning disability. In the case of people with intellectual disabilities, as a target population, we know that co-morbidities are common and may be missed due to diagnostic overshadowing. A diligent search should be carried out for a cause of a change in behaviour, and a careful history should include trying to identify whether the start was sudden or gradual, and when it occurred. The statement from a carer who knows the patient well should never be ignored and, despite the difficulties and extra time needed, a working diagnosis and treatment that best fits the facts should be agreed, with earlier review than usual, if the uncertainty justifies it. Caution is required if a patient has been under the care of a succession of support workers because he or she could have sustained an unnoticed injury. For example, if a patient suddenly stopped weight bearing, an X-ray of the lower limb might reveal an unexpected fracture. Many elderly PWID have osteoporosis.

Annual health checks

Following the introduction of annual health checks for adults with PWID in Wales,[3] the Department of Health in England introduced similar annual health checks in 2008 as a Directed Enhanced Service.[5] This allows the consideration perhaps of less obvious clinical problems in protected time and, for GP registrars, offers learning experience in engaging with people with intellectual disabilities and their carers. The evidence is that such structured comprehensive checks identify and therefore address twice as many health problems as standard primary care alone.[4]

At the last count, only 52% of those patients entitled in England actually received a check. This was the final complete cycle funded and supervised by Primary Care Trusts (PCTs).[10] The care of PWID is coming under the aegis of the new Clinical Commissioning Groups (CCGs), which have different boundaries, and cover different, larger areas from the PCTs. The Improving Health and Lives Learning Disabilities Observatory (IHAL) (now part of Public Health England), which has the responsibility for reporting the progress in the introduction of the annual health checks in England, may find it difficult to exactly compare 'like with like'.[11]

The monitoring of this has now passed to Public Health England.

It is to be hoped that the returns will show and increase towards the 90% target. Failure to improve should be seen as a population health inequality issue. As well as a responsibility for the CCG, at the patient level it is also the responsibility of practices to ensure they offer all adult patients on their learning disabilities register the opportunity for a comprehensive clinical check-up annually.

Where there is time to be fully comprehensive, the yield for some standard health parameters may be comparatively small, so it has been proposed that an annual health check for people with intellectual disabilities should concentrate on appropriate functional intellectual disability-specific health issues.[12] In Appendix B on p. 153 an example of an *aide-mémoire* grid shows how a check based on medical health function might look. Appendix C, on p. 154, shows a post-health check action plan.

Summary

The diagnosis of intellectual disability is associated with a variety of health inequalities, some of which are also inequities. Limited cognitive ability disadvantages the individual in many areas of life, including accessing and navigating health services. Carers advocate on behalf of people with intellectual disabilities, but the patient's doctor and primary care team also have a clear responsibility to make reasonable adjustments to meet their patients' individual clinical and other associated needs. This chapter suggests some ways in which this responsibility may be fulfilled.

Paired case scenarios

....

Case scenario 1: patients A and B

Two female patients, both aged 19, consult you.

....

Patient A

The first points to a very small, slightly inflamed 1 mm spot/papule on her cheek.

She asks if it could be cancer. You reassure. She requests treatment. You point out that it is so small that treatment, in your opinion, would be inappropriate and unsuccessful, and that given time the spot should become less obvious. She asks about excision. You point out that the scar from excision might be bigger and more trouble than the spot. She demands something be done about her spot, but you reiterate your opinion that no treatment, apart from observation, is necessary. She expresses her dissatisfaction and there is an impasse. She says that despite your reassurances she remains concerned about the spot and demands a second opinion. You eventually accede to her request.

....

Patient B

The second patient is shy and mumbles about the spots on her face; she has florid acne. You prescribe a skin cleanser, and advise her to return if it is not improving. She has Down's syndrome.

Reflect on these contrasting consultations from the perspective of:

- time taken
- patient/doctor control of agenda
- communication
- treatment outcome and follow-up.

In respect of the second patient, what changes could you make to reduce any health inequality gap within a routine surgery appointment?

Case scenario 2: patients C and D

Two patients present in your surgery, both males aged 65 with a two-month history of epigastric discomfort and symptoms suggestive of reflux, with no previous history of this complaint.

Patient C

Patient C is a bank manager. He is given a standard lifestyle leaflet, advised to continue OTC antacids and referred for endoscopy. He has this with biopsy, which turns out to be negative for H. pylori.

Some inflammation of pylorus is confirmed and he is commenced on a PPI.

The bank manager recovered after a period of temporary stress with the course of PPI. His endoscopy reassured him there was nothing serious and he did not need treatment for H. pylori.

Patient D

The second patient is brought by a paid carer. He lives in a residential care home, having recently moved from a long-stay hospital. He has moderate learning disability secondary to cerebral palsy. As he has not taken any antacids, 60 are prescribed on a p.r.n.* basis. Referral for endoscopy is considered but there are doubts whether he will be able to cooperate with the procedure or understand why it is being done. Lifestyle advice** is given, but as he is unable to read the carer is asked to explain this and to bring him back when and if he needs more antacids.

Three months later you get a letter from the local hospital saying he is being discharged after admission with a haematemesis. You review his medications and find that the antacid was not repeated.

....

* Patients in residential care on p.r.n. drugs are at risk of under-treatment. This is because the patient may have problems obtaining these when actually needed; carers tend to be cautious about giving drugs, even when these are prescribed for the patient.

** Dietary advice; postural advice including tilting up the head of the bed; stopping smoking.

In the case of patient D would referral for barium studies or investigation for evidence of past or active *H. pylori* infection have altered your treatment and the outcome?

The carer here has a pivotal role in ensuring that communication of diagnosis, investigation and treatment is carried out. Where the patient cannot take full responsibility for his health care additional responsibility partly falls on the carer. Does the GP need to take additional responsibility? How?

Consider whether in the case of the two patients with intellectual disabilities (B and D) attending an annual health check would have changed the way they were treated.[13]

References

1. Hart J T. The inverse care law. *Lancet* 1971; **1(7696)**: 405–12.

2. Scott-Samuel A. Health inequalities politics and policy under New Labour. Equity in Health Research and Development Unit, University of Liverpool, 2004, www.sochealth.co.uk/public-health-and-wellbeing/poverty-and-inequality/health-inequalities-politics-and-policy-under-new-labour/ [accessed October 2013].

3. Baxter H, Lowe K, Houston H, *et al*. Previously unidentified morbidity in patients with intellectual disability. *British Journal of General Practice* 2006; **56(523)**: 93–8.

4. Cooper S A, Morrison J, Melville C, *et al*. Improving the health of people with intellectual disabilities: outcomes of a health screening programme after 1 year. *Journal of Intellectual Disability Research* 2006; **50(9)**: 667–77.

5. Signpost Sheffield. Introduction to Direct Enhanced Services: Annual Health Checks for people with a learning disability. www.signpostsheffield.org.uk/Staying-healthy/gpcorner/desintro.html [accessed October 2013].

6. van Schrojenstein Lanteman-De Valk HMJ, Metsemakers JFM, Haveman MJ, *et al.* Health problems in people with intellectual disability in general practice: a comparative study. *Family Practice* 2000; **17(5)**: 405–7.

7. Disability Rights Commission. *Equal Treatment: closing the gap.* London: DRC, 2006, http://disability-studies.leeds.ac.uk/files/library/DRC-Health-FI-main.pdf   [accessed October 2013].

8. Harvey RF Gordon PC, Hadley N, *et al.* Effects of sleeping with the bed-head raised and of ranitidine in patients with severe peptic oesophagitis. *Lancet* 1987; **2(8569)**: 1200–3.

9. Kaltenbach T, Crockett S, Gerson LB. Are lifestyle measures effective in patients with gastroesophageal reflux disease? An evidence-based approach. *Archives of Internal Medicine* 2006; **166(9)**: 965–71.

10. Glover G, Emerson E, Evison F. *The Uptake of Health Checks for Adults with Learning Disabilities: 2008/9 to 2011/12.* IHAL, 2012, www.improvinghealthandlives.org.uk/uploads/doc/vid_16402_IHAL2012-07%20Health%20Checks%20for%20People%20with%20Learning%20Disabilities%202008-9%20to%202011-12v3.pdf   [accessed September 2013].

11. Glover G. 20130925 Glover Learning Disability Health Check Numbers 2012-3.pptx, 2013, www.improvinghealthandlives.org.uk/publications/1197/Health_checks_for_people_with_learning_disabilities_in_England,_2012/2013   [accessed October 2013].

12. Chauhan U, Kontopantelis E, Campbell S, *et al.* Health checks in primary care for adults with intellectual disabilities: how extensive should they be? *Journal of Intellectual Disability Research* 2010; **54(6)**: 479–86, doi: 1111/j.1365-2788.2010.01263.x.

13. Hoghton M. *A Step by Step Guide for GP Practices: annual health checks for people with learning disability.* London: RCGP, 2010.

Appendices

Appendix A: Learning disabilities pre-health check questionnaire

Please complete the following form and return in the stamped addressed envelope to the surgery. Circle your answers.

Name .... Date of birth ....

I want/do not want to come for a health check at the surgery on .... (date)

At .... (time of appointment offered)

If you do not want to receive any more appointments please say why ....

....

....

I want to come but cannot come on the date you offer; please send me a new appointment.

When I come I will be supported by a:

Paid carer ....

Family carer ....

Friend ....

Other person ....

I have problems attending the surgery due to:

Transport difficulties ....

Hearing impairment ....

Communication difficulties ....

I do not like waiting with other people ....

I do not like waiting a long time ....

Other reasons; please state ....

Important medical problems I want to discuss with you when I come are:

(please state what aspects of your health you wish to discuss with me)

1 ....

....

2 ....

....

3 ....

....

If you have difficulties with some of the above questions we can discuss them at your appointment or you may like to phone me on tel number .... at ....

.... Nurse/Doctor

Appendix B: *Aide-mémoire* of important clinical functions to be checked for all adults undergoing annual health review

(These are in addition to standard clinical parameters such as blood pressure, immunisations and specific associated conditions such as epilepsy and diabetes, and medication review. Visual function needs checking by an optician.)

Function	Assessment	Procedure
BMI	Weight/height tables	Diet and monitor
Weight change	Weight compared with weight at last year's check	If evidence of significant increase or decrease in weight (±5%), investigate and recommend diet adjustment and monitoring
Hearing impairment	Auriscopy/whisper test	Remove impacted cerumen; reassess hearing; ? refer for hearing aid
Swallowing/reflux	Enquire regarding dysphagia/dyspepsia, etc.; ? *H. pylori* check	Investigate and/or treat empirically, if appropriate. Advise head-up bed tilt
Bowel action	Enquire re. constipation/loose stools (using Bristol stool charts); ? continence status	Advise re. diet, and if necessary treat (causes)
Micturition	History/symptoms/urinalysis; continence/enuresis; dipstick/MSU	Further investigate, advise and treat as appropriate
Mobility	Enquire re. walking distance – decreasing? and wheelchair usage – increasing? Check re. posture	Address causes of reduction in ambulation. Consider physiotherapy and review walking aids
Mental state	Check for depression and enquire regarding significant life events	Use validated score system, such as PAS-ADD. Treat as required. Refer to specialist if necessary

Appendix C: Post-annual health check action plan

Tick in first column to indicate action required, and in second when completed.   ✓   ✓

Dear ....

(Name of patient/carer)

We found you were in good health and need not attend for another health check until next year

We recommend to following treatments/tests/actions

Book an appointment at this surgery for

Blood test

Urine test (bring sample)

Other test ....

Contact your doctor to discuss results .... days after test done

Make an appointment with the practice nurse ....
.... in .... days' time for

Weight check

Blood pressure check

Ear syringe

Other procedure ....

Contact the community learning disability team
(tel. no.) .... to make appointment
with ....

Community specialist LD nurse

Speech and language therapist

Social worker

Other professional ....

Arrange for an appointment with

Dentist

Optician

Dietician

Other ....

Expect a hospital appointment to see ....

Other actions ....
....
....

Signed .... Date ....

10 Adolescent health

Dick Churchill

Aim

Young people have traditionally been considered to be a relatively healthy group within the population. As a consequence they have often been marginalised in terms of health service provision. Although there have been some positive changes in recent years, some of the most disadvantaged and 'at risk' young people still do not receive the care that they need, with implications for long-term health inequalities. This chapter aims to describe some of the factors that make adolescents a unique group in society and some of the steps that can be taken to improve appropriate primary care health provision for them.

Key learning points

- Adopt a holistic approach to assessing adolescent development.

- Recognise the range of health issues that affect young people, how these can be inter related and how they can impact on future health inequalities.

- Describe approaches to improving primary care health services for young people.

- Discuss the impact of legal and ethical issues on the management of young people.

Introduction: adolescents in society

The World Health Organization defines adolescence chronologically as being between the ages of ten to 19, but it is generally more helpful to consider it as a developmental stage describing the period in life between the onset of physiologically normal puberty and the acceptance of adult identity and behaviour.[1,2] There are currently approximately 7.7 million adolescents aged ten to 19 living in the UK, constituting about 12% of the population.[3]

In contrast with many disadvantaged groups with whom health professionals may have little in common, every adult has personally experienced what it has been like to be an adolescent. Such knowledge may lead to a false sense of 'expertise' and paternalistic approaches that only serve to widen the gap between generations: we, as professionals, may purport to 'know' what it is like, while the young person with whom we are dealing is certain that their experience is unique and personal to them.

In society our perceptions about adolescence are shaped not only by own personal experiences, but also by the media. A Young Researcher Network in 2008 reported that the majority of press coverage about young people was negative or neutral, and there is a tendency for the press to sensationalise and exaggerate problems.[4] Since young people are relatively less able to respond to such criticism than other groups in society they are, as a group, left tainted by such negative stereotyping.

Adolescent development

The processes that take place during adolescence need to be considered holistically, as they encompass not only the physiological changes of puberty with associated psychological and emotional transition, but also externally mediated influences affecting the position and responsibilities of a young person within society. It is important to understand these transitions because they influence the ways both in which young people behave and also are perceived by others.

Puberty

The most outwardly apparent changes that occur during adolescence are those of the physical changes associated with puberty. Puberty is initiated in late childhood by a cascade of endocrine triggers that lead to sexual maturation and reproductive capability.[5] There is a growth spurt in both sexes associated with development of secondary sex characteristics and with the menarche in girls and with genital enlargement in boys.

There are wide variations in the timing of onset of puberty, but perceived deviations from the norm can be a significant cause of unspoken anxiety for many young people.[2] In boys the onset of the growth spurt is preceded by increase in testicular size and pubic hair growth that may occur any time between the ages of nine and 15. In girls the first visible change of puberty is the development of breast buds, which can occur as young as eight, but may not take place till 14 years of age.[6]

Neurobiological development

It was traditionally believed that the brain was fully developed by the end of childhood. However, modern imaging techniques have demonstrated that significant developments continue until much later in adolescence.[7,8] Such changes include synaptic 'pruning' (which reduces grey matter and increases cognitive efficiency), increased myelination (which speeds up nerve transmission dramatically in the affected areas) and increased density of dopaminergic neurotransmission.

Many of these changes occur in the pre-frontal cortex, which is responsible for such skills as priority setting, organisation, strategy formation, impulse control and attention allocation. Continuing neurobiological development therefore accounts directly for many of the cognitive and behavioural changes that are observed during the transition from childhood to adulthood.

Psychological development

Some key areas of psychosocial transition that take place during adolescence include the change from concrete to abstract thinking, increased awareness of the perceptions of others and the development of personal identity.[1,9]

Between the ages of 12 and adulthood young people develop the ability to think about hypothetical and imaginary events, adopt a hypothetico-deductive approach to problem solving, and assess multiple outcomes.[10] In the context of health care, a capacity for a degree of abstract thinking is vital for the ability to give informed consent for treatment, and for managing chronic illness regimens independently.[2]

In parallel with this, young people move from an egocentric belief that others share the same preoccupations and ideas as themselves towards an appreciation of other perspectives that they then incorporate into their own decision-making processes.[11,12]

One of the most important psychological tasks for a young person is that of developing his or her own personal identity in terms of self-concept and self-image.[13] This encompasses a whole range of factors including sexual orientation, ethnicity, personal 'tastes', beliefs and attitudes. However, the process of identity formation involves both experimentation and exploration before a commitment to continuing beliefs and behaviours is sustained. Young people who struggle to find their own identity tend to present as lacking confidence and with low self-esteem.

The social context

It is important to recognise that, while many of the behaviours and emotions of young people, such as sexual motivation, mood swings, experimentation and impulsiveness, can be explained in neurophysiological terms, they are modified by the social environment and context in which a young person is developing.

Adolescence as we know it today in the UK is heavily influenced by the social and economic culture in which we live. The lives of young people today are barely recognisable compared with those of even a generation ago, and equally there are marked differences between the process of adolescence in Western society and that in developing countries.[1]

Key influences include the transition from education to employment, family structures and the legal framework. Increased opportunities for continuing education or training beyond school mean that financial independence is delayed. Consequently young people tend to live at home for longer and the process of completing adolescence is delayed. Increased divorce rates in the UK have resulted in a much higher proportion of young people living in lone-parent or reconstituted families in which the relationships and parenting roles are not clearly defined, and so young people rely more on peer support and friendships. Finally, the legislative system dictates the age at which young people are permitted to develop autonomy in certain areas.

Another key difficulty for young people in society is 'the lack of recognition of them as distinctly different from children as well as adults' such that they can be 'a "forgotten group" caught between child and adult, and therefore between bureaucratic barriers and professional spheres of influence'.[14]

....

Case scenario 1

Laura, aged 11, was taken to see the GP by her mum because of 'behaviour problems'. Her mother described oppositional behaviour and low mood lasting several months. However, her school performance seemed unaffected. An exploration of the social situation revealed that Laura and her mum were living with her grandparents following an acrimonious separation from her father. Laura was sharing a bedroom with her older sister who hated her father for what had happened. Laura, on the other hand, had sympathy for her father.

Although relatively obvious to an objective outside observer, Laura's family had failed to appreciate the emotional consequences of such strained relationships on Laura. Dysfunctional family relationships are a frequent factor in exacerbating normal psychological reactions during adolescence.

....

Young people and their health

Although mortality rates are relatively low amongst adolescents, they begin to increase from the age of 15, with the commonest causes of death being injury, poisoning and road traffic accidents, and with rates being significantly higher in males than females.[3] In addition, while young people might otherwise generally be considered a healthy population, they can adopt attitudes, actions and behaviours that can have long-term effects on their health. In his 2007 report the Chief Medical Officer for England acknowledged that 'the effects of poor health during the teenage years can last a lifetime. Keeping adolescents healthy is a valuable investment in the nation's future.'[15] One obvious example is that most people who start smoking cigarettes do so in their early teens but, if the behaviour is sustained, it is likely to result in a significantly reduced life expectancy due to lung cancer or cardiovascular disease in the long term.[16]

The areas of greatest concern at a public health level relate to young people's sexual and reproductive health, mental health and the adoption of potentially harmful health-related behaviours such as smoking, alcohol and substance misuse. Although these are often considered separately, health risks tend to cluster such that the most disadvantaged young people are vulnerable to a whole range of adverse health outcomes (see Box 10.1). It is therefore important that primary care health professionals are equipped to adopt a holistic approach in the management of young people so that they can help them deal with the whole spectrum of problems that they may experience, rather than focus on single issues in isolation, such as contraception.

While the remainder of this chapter focuses on two of the most important public health areas of teenage health, those of sexual health and

---

Box 10.1 Young people and vulnerability

Young people in the following categories are at a higher risk of a range of disadvantages and health problems, including teenage pregnancy, sexually transmitted diseases, alcohol and substance misuse, accidents, emotional and mental health problems, and self-harm. The list is not exclusive and many factors are interrelated. However, it is also important to recognise that young people who are exposed to adverse circumstances do not inevitably experience adverse outcomes.

- Living in socially disadvantaged families (often associated with low income, lone parenthood, parental unemployment, etc.).

- Long-term parental discord and family conflict.

- Living in care.

- History of physical, emotional or sexual abuse, or neglect.

- Low educational attainment or school exclusion.

- Close family history of mental illness or alcohol/substance misuse.

- Youth offending.

- Chronic illness, or personal alcohol or substance misuse.

- Early-onset sexual activity.

mental health, it is important to recognise that young people often have their own specific concerns that need to be acknowledged and addressed, however minor they might appear to an adult clinician. Some of the likely concerns have been identified from analysis of emails sent to an online website for young people, and the most frequent questions were about sex, relationships and body parts.[17] There are also other problems such as obesity and eating disorders, which are not discussed further in this chapter, but which are highly relevant to an adolescent population.

Another group of young people who merit special consideration are those with disability or long-term or life-limiting conditions, especially at the stage of transition between paediatric and adult specialist services. This can be a difficult experience, particularly for those who have had a high level of care as children, often with extensive parental involvement, when many of their primary care needs may have been addressed by a specialist team. General practice may need to play a greater role in the lives of such young people as they enter adult care, and two important areas are those of negotiating increased autonomy from their parents, and also addressing their holistic health needs, not only those related specifically to their condition.

Sexual and reproductive health issues

Sexual maturation is a normal part of adolescent development. However, the onset of sexual activity is associated with multiple health risks, the two most important being unintended pregnancy in girls and sexually transmitted infections in either sex.

In recent years the UK has had one of the highest teenage pregnancy rates in Western Europe. While there has been a significant fall in the under-18 conception rate in England and Wales, from 47.1 per thousand in 1969 to 30.9 per thousand in 2011, there are still significant regional variations and approximately 50% of pregnancies end in abortion.[18] Alongside high teenage pregnancy rates there was a threefold increase in new diagnoses of Chlamydia infection since the 1990s, with the greatest increases being in young people under the age of 25.[19] While some of this may be due to increased detection of asymptomatic disease, much of the increase is due to higher rates of infection. Genital warts and genital herpes are also increasingly common among young people.

Several factors may have contributed to these trends. The age of onset of sexual activity has fallen dramatically over the past four decades, such that approximately one-third of young people now report having had sexual intercourse by the age of 16.[3,20] Early onset of sexual activity is associated with reduced contraceptive use, increased risk of teenage pregnancy and short duration of relationships.[21-23] There is also an increasing trend towards multiple partners, with one-fifth of 16–24-year-olds reporting having had ten or more sexual partners and a similar proportion reporting having concurrent partners.[24]

Clearly not all teenage pregnancies are unintended, and some can be a positive experience.[24-28] However, teenage pregnancy is generally associated with increased risks to both the mother and child in terms of both physical and psychosocial outcomes.[29-31] In addition, teenage mothers are more likely to be socially disadvantaged because of unemployment and reduced life chances, and to have significantly higher levels of mental illness following childbirth.[32,33] Children of teenage mothers have higher levels of mortality and morbidity. They are specifically at increased risk of sudden infant death syndrome, and of both accidental and non-accidental injury.[30,34] In the long term they are more likely to have behavioural problems,[35] have lower levels of educational attainment and a higher risk of economic inactivity.[33] They are also more likely to become teenage parents themselves, so that the cycle of disadvantage is perpetuated.

There are wide regional and local variations in the rates of teenage pregnancy and sexually transmitted infections. Some of the key risk factors are socioeconomic deprivation, living in care, early onset of sexual activity, low educational attainment and expectations, truancy, having a mother who was also a teen parent, and drug and alcohol misuse.[36-43]

While there are clearly social determinants of sexual activity and sexual health that are beyond the scope of health service providers, a recent review suggests that good relationship/sex education, linked with accessible contraception and sexual health advice, is the most effective method of reducing teenage pregnancy rates.[44,45] General practices are a key provider of contraceptive services[46-48] but have been criticised for not being sufficiently accessible for young people. In addition young people have not always been aware that they can access general practice for sexual health advice.[49,50] These issues are discussed further later on in this chapter. However, the encouragement that GPs have received to promote the use of long-acting reversible contraception (LARC), within the Quality and Outcomes Framework of the GMS contract, may already have had an impact on conception rates in young people.

....

Case scenario 2

Sarah, aged 17, came in to see a GP a few days after Christmas to request emergency contraception. It was apparent from her records that she had previously been prescribed the oral contraceptive pill. However, Sarah said that she had stopped it a few weeks previously when she split up with her boyfriend because he was sleeping with someone else. However, they had got back together at Christmas and had slept together a few times but she hadn't used any protection because they were drunk.

A simple request for contraception can become much more complicated once the background is explored. Not only is simple emergency contraception unlikely to be appropriate here, but also Sarah seems unaware of her risk of acquiring sexually transmitted infection. Oral contraception is unreliable in young people who stop and start it in reaction to the status of their current relationship, which is why LARC is often a more suitable alternative.

Mental health issues

Variations in mood and temporary 'deviant' behaviours are part of the normal adolescent process.[51] Mental health problems represent a spectrum of divergence from normal mental health that can range from experiencing relatively minor symptoms or difficulties, through to disorders involving a marked deviation from normality, together with impaired personal functioning or development, or significant suffering, and finally to more severe forms of mental illness such as depression or schizophrenia.[52]

The potential impact of mental health problems in young people were clearly highlighted in the *National Service Framework for Children, Young People and Maternity Services*:

> Mental health problems in children [and young people] are associated with educational failure, family disruption, disability, offending and antisocial behaviour, placing demands on social services, schools and the youth justice system. Untreated mental health problems create distress not only in the children and young people, but also for their families and carers, continuing into adult life, and affecting the next generation.[53]

The majority of life-long mental health problems begin in adolescence with approximately half starting by the mid-teens, and three-quarters by the mid-twenties. Later onsets develop mostly as secondary conditions.[54] Moreover, adults who experience mental health problems in youth are significantly more likely to have lower incomes and less likely to be in stable relationships in later life.[55] The long-term health outcomes for young people developing severe mental illness are particularly poor, with a two-to fourfold increased risk of premature death and average life expectancy shortened by ten years.[56] Some young people are more likely to develop emotional and mental health problems than others. This is related to the balance between factors that appear to enhance vulnerability and those that are protective and promote resilience, or the ability to cope in the face of adverse situations and events.[57]

The spectrum of mental and emotional health disorders in young people ranges from mild depression and anxiety states to severe psychotic illness, eating disorders and significant self-harm and suicide. Suicide rates are about three times greater in young men aged 15 to 24 than in young women at approximately 13 per 100,000.[20] However, self-harming is much more common to the extent that it can be considered as a maladaptive response to emotional pain, rather than a mental health disorder in itself. Self-harming behaviour can include cutting, burning, hair pulling and ingesting substances including overdosing. An inquiry into self-harm in young people by the Mental Health Foundation and Camelot Foundation concluded that the incidence of self-cutting was between 1 in 12 and 1 in 15 but only a small proportion of such incidences ever come to the attention of medical services or even family members.[58]

In cross-sectional surveys nearly 1 in 10 children and young people have been shown to have a clinically diagnosable mental health disorder in the UK[59] but even higher rates (between 32% and 38%) have been found among primary care attenders.[60-62] The commonest classifiable mental health disorders in adolescents are depression (3–5%), anxiety (4–6%), attention deficit/hyperactivity disorder (2–4%), eating disorders (1–2%), conduct disorders (4–6%) and substance misuse disorders (2–3%).[51] Conduct disorders were more common than emotional disorders overall, and specifically among boys compared with girls. Emotional disorders were most common in older girls.

Young people with mental health problems may present to their GP with recurrent physical symptoms or their parents may bring them because of behavioural problems, but explicit presentations with emotional symptoms are uncommon.[63] This may be one of the reasons why the detection rate of such problems by GPs is less then 25%.[60,64] However, other reasons may include reluctance on the part of GPs to diagnose problems for which they feel relatively unskilled to help, or the perception that most such problems are transient.[65]

Mental health problems are more likely to be detected if some of the consultation is spent briefly exploring psychosocial issues. One framework for enquiry is the use of HEADSS: Home; Education; Activities; Drugs; Sex; Self-Harm.[66] Consultations with young people tend to be shorter than those with adults,[67] and simply allowing more time exploring psychosocial issues is likely to result in a greater yield. If a problem is identified then it is important to assess its severity and plan an appropriate management strategy, which may range from simple supportive 'watchful waiting' in the case of emotional distress, to prompt referral if there are suspicions of early psychosis or risk of serious self-harm.[65]

Youth-friendly primary care

In the past 20 years numerous research studies have explored the attitudes of young people to primary care and the perceived barriers to accessing such care. Concerns about confidentiality are always most dominant[50,68–71] but other concerns include embarrassment, difficulties in getting appointments, and the negative attitudes of GPs and staff.[50,68,72] Young people consider it important to have a GP who is interested in teenage problems, and also the option to choose between a male and female healthcare professional;[63] indeed, there is some evidence that such provision increases the uptake of contraceptive care and can have an impact on teenage pregnancy rates.[36]

Over the years many general practices have experimented with providing enhanced services for young people, for example by inviting them for specific health checks. There has been limited evaluation of such approaches, and the results have been very mixed.[73–77] However, in response to the concerns raised by young people, the RCGP Adolescent Working Party launched a campaign entitled 'Getting it Right for Young People in General Practice' in the early 2000s to encourage all practices to take some small steps to providing better care for teenagers. Some of the concepts from this campaign were more recently adopted by the Department of Health in designing a package called 'You're Welcome', which consists of a series of quality criteria by which health providers can be judged for their 'youth friendliness'.[78] The areas covered within 'You're Welcome' are shown in Box 10.2.

In practical terms, general practices who are seeking to provide improved services for the young people registered with them need to consider both general principles and the specific local needs of the population.[79] For example, young people will only be able to use a service if it is accessible to them, both in location and time. A practice that has a surgery next to a school or college may be able to provide appointments at lunchtimes or after school, while a rural practice whose young people have to travel to school or college may need to offer later appointments or even consider setting up an outreach service within the educational establishment. Involving young people in planning is essential when considering offering focused services, but their views should also be included when evaluating existing services such as when carrying out patient satisfaction surveys.

While initiatives such as 'You're Welcome' seek to promote services young people will feel more comfortable in attending, the impact of inter-

> **Box 10.2 Areas covered in the Department of Health's 'You're Welcome' criteria for youth-friendly health services**
>
> - Accessibility.
> - Publicity.
> - Confidentiality & Consent.
> - The Environment.
> - Staff Training, Attitudes, Skills and Values.
> - Joined-up Working.
> - Monitoring & Evaluation, and Involvement of Young People.
> - Health Issues for Adolescents.
> - Specific Criteria for Sexual Health and Child & Adolescent Mental Health Services.

personal communication between the clinician and the young person should not be underestimated. Here are some examples of quotes from young people about their perceptions:[80]

- 'I'm really intimidated when I go to my doctor … I sit there: "Yes doctor, no doctor."'

- 'You've got to put on such an act, and you're only in there for five minutes!'

- 'It's not that he doesn't listen … sometimes he doesn't fully comprehend that he's talking in a way you can't understand.'

Few health professionals in primary care have received specific training in how best to communicate with young people, and in fact they sometimes report feeling 'uncomfortable' when dealing with teenage problems.[81] Recently, training packages such as the 'HEAR' DVDs (RCGP Adolescent Health Group, 2008 and 2012) and the E-Learning for Healthcare Adolescent Health Project have been produced to improve the confidence of clinicians both in communication and clinical aspects of teenage health. More details are provided at the end of this chapter.

Finally, it is important to consider different ways of communicating with young people. This is a generation who are used to mobile communication by phone, the internet and on smart devices, and may often be more comfortable communicating by these means rather than face to face, especially for sensitive issues.[82] General practice needs to be pre-pared to innovate and to explore the use of new technologies if it is to keep in touch with the new generation.

Legal and ethical issues

There has historically been some confusion about the rights of young people to consult independently, to consent to treatment, and to have information about them kept confidential, especially if they are aged under 16.[83-85] This is because, in practice, there is a balance to be achieved between promoting autonomy and safeguarding. Such confusion is proba-bly one of the factors that has contributed to young people's concerns about confidentiality in general practice discussed previously. The General Medi-cal Council has produced clear guidance for doctors on these issues,[2,86] although ethical dilemmas will still occur, and individual clinicians need to be able to make informed judgements about individual circumstances.

Below is a summary of general principles.

- There is no absolute lower age limit at which a young person can consult a GP independently. The same duty of confidentiality applies to consultations with young people as to those with adults.

- Any decision to offer treatment to a young person under the age of 16 without parental consent should be based on the Fraser Guidelines (see Box 10.3). Strictly speaking the term 'Fraser competence' applies only to the field of contraception, whereas the term 'Gillick competence' is not limited to sexual health and applies more broadly to issues of consent in under-16s. The key component is the capacity of a young person to consent in his or her own right, and this depends on both the young person's developmental stage and the treatment or intervention being considered.

- There are specific circumstances in which disclosure of information may be necessary, such as for safeguarding purposes, but even in such circumstances every effort should be made to gain the consent of the young person to make the disclosure and they should be fully informed of the disclosure and the reasons for it.

- There are some specific variations in the law relating to young people between different countries in the UK.

Box 10.3 **The Fraser Guidelines**

Although these guidelines were based on a ruling about general practice prescribing of the oral contraceptive pill without parental consent, they are often now accepted as applying more broadly.

A young person is competent to consent to contraceptive advice or treatment if:

- the young person understands the doctor's advice

- the doctor cannot persuade the young person to inform his or her parents, or allow the doctor to inform them

- the young person is very likely to begin or to continue having sexual intercourse with or without contraceptive treatment

- unless he or she receives contraceptive advice or treatment, the young person's physical or mental health, or both, are likely to suffer

- the young person's best interests require the doctor to give contraceptive advice, treatment or both without parental consent.

A full discussion of the legal and ethical issues is beyond the scope of this chapter, but clinicians who work with young people need to be fully conversant with both safeguarding principles and the rights of young people.

....

Case scenario 3

After much persuasion, and repeated consultations, Martin, a 14-year-old, was eventually persuaded by his GP to go and see the counsellor at the local youth clinic about the problems that he was having in dealing with anger. During the first assessment visit Martin disclosed that he had seen his dad hit his mother a few months earlier. The counsellor decided to notify social services against Martin's wishes and this caused significant upheaval at home, with no eventual action taken. Martin never returned to see the counsellor.

Young people cite fear of a breach of confidentiality as the greatest barrier to seeking help from health professionals. Confidentiality policies do not impress them – instead 'trust' is much more dependent on interpersonal relationships and effective communication. It often takes time to build. However, once trust is established then it is possible to discuss disclosure of information, with the young person understanding that such a suggestion is, at least, being made in his or her best interest.

....

Conclusion

Young people's health poses a real challenge to primary care clinicians. However, many of the main barriers to effective care are related to attitudes, understanding and communication. From the perspective of a young person, the most effective clinician is one that he or she can trust.

Useful resources

- Adolescent Health E-Learning Package, www.e-lfh.org.uk/projects/adolescent-health [a training package for all health professionals who deal with young people].

- The Association for Young People's Health (AYPH) is an organisation that was established to support and inform health professionals working with young people. Accessible via www.youngpeopleshealth.org.uk, it provides access to a number of resources.

- Department of Health. *Quality Criteria for Young People Friendly Health Services* (You're Welcome). London: DH, 2011, www.gov.uk/government/uploads/system/uploads/attachment_data/file/216350/dh_127632.pdf [accessed October 2013].

- HEAR: Helping Establish Adolescent Rapport (RCGP Adolescent Task Group, 2008) and HEAR-2 (RCGP Adolescent Health Group and Charlie Waller Memorial Trust, 2012): two DVDs designed to facilitate discussion about consultations between GPs and young people. Available from mailings@rcgpacps.org.

- Youth Health Talk, www.youthhealthtalk.org [a website about young people's real-life experiences of health and lifestyle].

References

1. Coleman J C, Hendry L B. The nature of adolescence. In: J C Coleman (ed.). *Adolescence and Society* (3rd edn). London: Routledge, 1999, pp. 2–21.

2. Christie D, Viner R. Adolescent development. *British Medical Journal* 2005; **330(7486)**: 301–4.

3. Coleman J, Schofield J. *Key Data on Adolescence* (6th edn). Brighton: Trust for the Study of Adolescence, 2007.

4. Young Researcher Network. *Media Portrayal of Young People: impact and influences*. Leicester: National Youth Agency, 2008.

5. Patton G C, Viner R. Adolescent health 1: pubertal transitions in health. *Lancet* 2007; **369(9567)**: 1130–9.

6. Tanner J. Adolescent growth spurt. In: R Lerner, AC Petersen, J Brooks-Gunn (eds). *Encyclopedia of Adolescence (Volume 1)*. New York: Garland Publishing, 1991.

7. Ernst M, Mueller S C. The adolescent brain: insights from functional neuroimaging research. *Developmental Neurobiology* 2008; **68(6)**: 729–43.

8. Casey B J, Jones R M, Hare T A. The adolescent brain. *Annals of the New York Academy of Sciences* 2008; **1124**: 111–26.

9. Heaven P C L. *The Social Psychology of Adolescence* (2nd edn). Basingstoke, Hampshire: Palgrave, 2001.

10. Inhelder B, Piaget J. *The Growth of Logical Thinking*. London: Routledge & Kegan Paul, 1958.

11. Elkind D. Egocentrism in adolescence. *Child Development* 1967; **38(4)**: 1025–34.

12. Selman R L. Structural-developmental model of social cognition: implications for intervention research. *Counseling Psychologist* 1977; **6(4)**: 3–6.

13. Erikson E. *Identity, Youth and Crisis*. New York: W.W. Norton & Company, 1968.

14. Kennedy I. *Getting it Right for Children and Young People: overcoming cultural barriers in the NHS so as to meet their needs*. London: DH, 2010.

15. Donaldson L. *On the State of Public Health: annual report of the Chief Medical Officer 2007*. London: DH, 2008.

16. Holland W W, Fitzsimons B. Smoking in children. *Archives of Disease in Childhood* 1991; **66(11)**: 1269–70.

17. Aldolphs S, Mullany L, Smith C, *et al. Am I Normal? What adolescents want to know about health*. Nottingham: University of Nottingham, 2012.

18. Office for National Statistics. Conception statistics, England and Wales, 2011. 2013. www.ons.gov.uk/ons/rel/vsob1/conception-statistics--england-and-wales/2011/index.html [accessed August 2013].

19. Health Protection Agency. *Diagnoses of Selected STIs by Strategic Health Authority, Country, Sex and Age Group, United Kingdom: 1997–2006*. London: HPA, 2007.

20. Hagell A, Coleman J, Brooks F. *Key Data on Adolescence 2013*. London, AYPH, 2013.

21. Mellanby A, Phelps F, Tripp J H. Teenagers, sex, and risk-taking. *British Medical Journal* 1993; **307(6895)**: 25.

22. Churchill D, Allen J, Pringle M, *et al*. Teenagers at risk of unintended pregnancy: identification of practical risk markers for use in general practice from a retrospective analysis of case records in the United Kingdom. *International Journal of Adolescent Medicine & Health* 2002; **14(2)**: 153–60.

23. Wellings F, Nanchahal K, Macdowall W, *et al*. Sexual behaviour in Britain: early heterosexual experience. *Lancet* 2001; **358(9296)**: 1843–50.

24. Johnson A M, Mercer C H, Erens B, *et al*. Sexual behaviour in Britain: partnerships, practices, and HIV risk behaviours. *Lancet* 2001; **358(9296)**: 1835–42.

25. Henshaw S K. Unintended pregnancy in the United States. *Family Planning Perspectives* 1998; **30(1)**: 24–9, 46.

26. Kiernan K. *Transition to Parenthood: young mothers, young fathers – associated factors and later life experiences*. London: LSE, 1995.

27. Lee E, Clements S, Ingham R, *et al. A Matter of Choice? Explaining national variation in teenage abortion and motherhood*. York: Joseph Rowntree Foundation, 2004.

28. Seamark C J, Lings P. Positive experiences of teenage motherhood: a qualitative study. *British Journal of General Practice* 2004; **54(508)**: 813–18.

29. Jacobson L D, Wilkinson C, Pill R. Teenage pregnancy in the United Kingdom in the 1990s: the implications for primary care. *Family Practice* 1995; **12(2)**: 232–6.

30. Irvine H, Bradley T, Cupples M, *et al*. The implications of teenage pregnancy and motherhood for primary health care: unresolved issues. *British Journal of General Practice* 1997; **47 (418)**: 323–6.

31. NHS Centre for Reviews and Dissemination. Preventing and reducing the adverse effects of unintended teenage pregnancies. *Effective Health Care* 1997; **3 (1)**: 1–12.

32. McIlroy C, Bradley T, Wilson-Davis K. Teenage parenthood and health: a pilot study. *Maternal & Child Health* 1995; **20**: 374–6.

33. Teenage Pregnancy Unit. Long-term consequences of teenage births for parents and their children. *Teenage Pregnancy Research Programme Research Briefing* 2004; **1**: 1–4.

34. Ekeus C, Christensson K, Hjern A. Unintentional and violent injuries among pre-school children of teenage mothers in Sweden: a national cohort study. *Journal of Epidemiology & Community Health* 2004; **58 (8)**: 680–5.

35. Trautmann-Vilalba, Gerhold M, Laucht M, *et al*. Early motherhood and disruptive behaviour in the school-age child. *Acta Paediatrica* 2004; **93 (1)**: 120–5.

36. Bethea J. *Teenage Pregnancy in Trent: factors associated with variations in rates and outcomes*. Nottingham: University of Nottingham, 2005.

37. Smith T. Influence of socioeconomic-factors on attaining targets for reducing teenage pregnancies. *British Medical Journal* 1993; **306 (6887)**: 1232–5.

38. Babb P. Teenage conceptions and fertility in England and Wales 1971–1991. *Population Trends* 2003; **74**: 12–17.

39. McLeod A. Changing patterns of teenage pregnancy: population based study of small areas. *British Medical Journal* 2001; **323 (7306)**: 199–203.

40. Seamark C J, Gray D J P. Like mother, like daughter: a general practice study of maternal influences on teenage pregnancy. *British Journal of General Practice* 1997; **47 (416)**: 175–6.

41. Holtgrave D R, Crosby R A. Social capital, poverty, and income inequality as predictors of gonorrhoea, syphilis, chlamydia and AIDS case rates in the United States. *Sexually Transmitted Infections* 2003; **79 (1)**: 62–4.

42. McPherson A, Macfarlane A. Contraception in general practice before teenage pregnancy: ambition may be best contraception. *British Medical Journal* 2001; **322 (7282)**: 363.

43. Stephenson J M, Stephenson J M, Strange V, *et al*. Pupil-led sex education in England (RIPPLE study): cluster-randomised intervention trial. *Lancet* 2004; **364 (9431)**: 338–46.

44. Kirby D. *Emerging Answers 2007: research findings on programs to reduce teen pregnancy and sexually transmitted diseases*. Washington, DC: National Campaign to Prevent Teen and Unplanned Pregnancy, 2007.

45. Department for Education and Skills. *Teenage Pregnancy Next Steps: guidance for local authorities and Primary Care Trusts on effective delivery of local strategies*. London: DfES, 2006.

46. Churchill D, Allen J, Pringle M, *et al*. Consultation patterns and provision of contraception in general practice before teenage pregnancy: case-control study. *British Medical Journal* 2000; **321 (7259)**: 486–9.

47. Seamark C J. More teenagers seem to be seeking contraceptive advice from their general practitioner. *British Medical Journal* 1997; **314 (7096)**: 1760.

48. Seamark C J, Pereira Gray D J. Do teenagers consult general practitioners for contraceptive advice? *British Journal of Family Planning* 1995; **21 (2)**: 50–1.

49. Balding J. *Young People into 2006*. Exeter: Schools Health Education Unit, 2006.

50. Burack R. Young teenagers' attitudes towards general practitioners and their provision of sexual health care. *British Journal of General Practice* 2000; **50(456)**: 550–4.

51. Michaud P A, Fombonne E. Common mental health problems. *British Medical Journal* 2005; **330(7495)**: 83–8.

52. British Medical Association, *Growing up in Britain: ensuring a healthy future for our children. A study of 0–5 year olds*. London: BMA, 1999.

53. Department of Health. *National Service Framework for Children, Young People and Maternity Services: the mental health and psychological well-being of children and young people*. London: DH, 2004.

54. Kessler R C, Amminger G P, Aguilar-Gaxiola S, *et al*. Age of onset of mental disorders: a review of recent literature. *Current Opinion In Psychiatry* 2007; **20(4)**: 359–64.

55. Goodman A, Joyce R, Smith J P. The long shadow cast by childhood physical and mental problems on adult life. *Proceedings of the National Academy of Sciences of the United States of America* 2011; **108(15)**: 6032–7.

56. Connolly M, Kelly C. Lifestyle and physical health in schizophrenia. *Advances in Psychiatric Treatment* 2005; **11**: 125–32.

57. Rutter M. Implications of resilience concepts for scientific understanding. *Annals of the New York Academy of Sciences* 2006; **1094**: 1–12.

58. Mental Health Foundation, Camelot Foundation. *Truth Hurts: report of the National Inquiry into Self-Harm among Young People*. London: Mental Health Foundation, 2006.

59. Green H, McGinnity A, Meltzer H, *et al*. *Mental Health of Children and Young People in Great Britain, 2004: summary report*. London: Palgrave Macmillan, 2005.

60. Kramer T, Garralda M E. Psychiatric disorders in adolescents in primary care. *British Journal of Psychiatry* 1998; **173**: 508–13.

61. Martinez R, Reynolds S, Howe A. Factors that influence the detection of psychological problems in adolescents attending general practices. *British Journal of General Practice* 2006; **56(529)**: 594–9.

62. Yates P, Kramer T, Garralda E. Depressive symptoms amongst adolescent primary care attenders: levels and associations. *Social Psychiatry and Psychiatric Epidemiology* 2004; **39(7)**: 588–94.

63. Churchill R, Allen J, Denman S, *et al*. Do the attitudes and beliefs of young teenagers towards general practice influence actual consultation behaviour? *British Journal of General Practice* 2000; **50(461)**: 953–7.

64. Sayal K, Taylor E. Detection of child mental health disorders by general practitioners. *British Journal of General Practice* 2004; **54(502)**: 348–52.

65. Churchill D. Child and adolescent mental health. In: A Cohen (ed.). *Delivering Mental Health in Primary Care: an evidence based approach*. London: RCGP, 2008, pp. 157–84.

66. McCabe R. Psychiatric disturbance. *Practitioner* 1992; **236**: 1150–4.

67. Jacobson L D, Owen P A. Study of teenage care in one general practice. *British Journal of General Practice* 1993; **43(373)**: 349.

68. Oppong-Odiseng A C K, Heycock E G. Adolescent health services: through their eyes. *Archives of Disease in Childhood* 1997; **77(2)**: 115–19.

69. McPherson A, Macfarlane A, Allen J. What do young people want from their GP? *British Journal of General Practice* 1996; **46(411)**: 627.

70. Hine A, Oakeshott P. Health services can be cool: partnership with adolescents in primary care. *Family Practice* 2001; **18(4)**: 462.

71. Davies L, Casey S. The adolescent view of accessing health services. *British Journal of General Practice* 1999; **49(443)**: 486–7.

72. Kari J, Donovan C, Li J, *et al.* Adolescents' attitudes to general practice in North London. *British Journal of General Practice* 1997; **47(415)**: 109–10.

73. Campbell A, Edgar S. Teenage screening in a general practice setting. *Health Visitor* 1993; **66(10)**: 365–6.

74. Cowap N. GPs need to be more proactive in providing health care to teenagers. *British Medical Journal* 1996; **313(7062)**: 941.

75. Donovan C, McCarthy S. Is there a place for adolescent screening in general practice? *Health Trends* 1988; **20**: 64.

76. Hibble A, Elwood J. Health promotion for young people. *Practitioner* 1992; **236**: 1140–3.

77. Walker Z, Townsend J, Oakley L, *et al.* Health promotion for adolescents in primary care: randomised controlled trial. *British Medical Journal* 2002; **325(7363)**: 524–7.

78. Department of Health. *Quality Criteria for Young People Friendly Health Services* (You're Welcome). London: DH, 2011, www.gov.uk/government/uploads/system/uploads/attachment_data/file/216350/dh_127632.pdf [accessed October 2013].

79. Churchill D, McPherson A. Getting it right in primary care: creating a child and young person friendly environment. In: R Chambers, K Licence (eds). *Looking after Children in Primary Care*. Oxford: Radcliffe, 2005, pp. 20–8.

80. Donovan C. *Bridging the Gap: a descriptive study of communication with teenagers in general practice*. Cardiff: Health Promotion Wales, 2001.

81. Donovan C, Suckling H. *Difficult Consultations with Adolescents*. Oxford: Radcliffe Medical Press, 2004.

82. Harvey K, Churchill D, Crawford P, *et al.* Health communication and adolescents: what do their emails tell us? *Family Practice* 2008; **25(4)**: 304–11.

83. Garside R, Ayres R, Owen M R, *et al.* General practitioners' attitudes to sexual activity in under-sixteens. *Journal of the Royal Society of Medicine* 2000; **93(11)**: 563–4.

84. Graham A, Moore L, Sharp D. Provision of emergency contraception in general practice and confidentiality for the under 16's: results of a postal survey by general practitioners in Avon. *Journal of Family Planning & Reproductive Health Care* 2001; **27(4)**: 193–6.

85. Sengupta S, Van Teijlingen E R, Smith B H. GPs, schoolgirls and sex: a cross cultural background comparison of general practitioner attitudes towards contraceptive service provision for young adolescent females in Scotland. *British Journal of Family Planning* 1998; **24(2)**: 39–42.

86. General Medical Council. *0–18 Years: guidance for all doctors*. London: GMC, 2007.

11 Clinical care of disadvantaged groups in remote and rural areas

A. Gordon Baird

Aim

The aim of this chapter is to help the reader to identify and manage factors that adversely affect health care in remote and rural areas. Health outcomes are poorer in rural areas. Deprivation is hidden because indices of deprivation have been designed primarily for use in urban settings and when applied to a rural setting fail to identify affected individuals or groups. The combination of these two factors and the scarcity or absence of other services means that the primary care team must be more flexible and develop a wider range of individual skills than urban counterparts. Living within a small community has advantages and disadvantages.

Key learning points

- In rural and remote communities, healthcare delivery differs from urban in a number of ways.

- Rural socioeconomic disadvantage is underestimated.

- Being rural or remote results in healthcare deprivation independent of socioeconomic factors.

- Mixtures of socioeconomic deprivation and rurality compound healthcare deficiencies.

- Solutions to disadvantages lie within primary care.

- The rural practitioner needs to develop skills and attitudes in addition to the generic skills within the GP curriculum.

Introduction

A fifth of the population of England and a third of the population of Scotland live in rural areas.[1] Wales and Northern Ireland lie somewhere between. For the purposes of measuring health or socioeconomic parameters, rural communities often find themselves included with urban areas. Even when urban areas are not included, the tools used to measure deprivation may fail to identify areas where socioeconomic deprivation exists.

Most measurement tools have been designed to examine urban areas of high homogeneous population density without the marked heterogeneity that characterises rural communities. As a result, little attention is paid to the effects of poverty in rural areas. The need to travel affects access to health care, both emergency and routine. Distance to services creates a barrier that negatively affects healthcare outcomes for the whole population. For example, car ownership is used as a marker for deprivation. In a rural and remote setting, even for those on subsistence income personal transport may be essential. For those disadvantaged, either in health or wealth, or affected by both, primary care needs to deliver care locally. In order to achieve this, the GP must take on a greater advocacy role and coordinate the link between health and social care more effectively using innovative solutions. Policymakers regularly ignore rural issues when formulating strategy[2] and should protect currently effective mechanisms that reduce these inequalities, e.g. local surgeries, community hospitals, dispensing, pre-hospital care. In England there has been criticism of funding for rural NHS trusts based on historical need.[3]

The demographics of an area may be defined in a way that fails to recognise small pockets of quite severe deprivation. The 'rural idyll', where a community is largely populated with commuters and retired professionals, invariably hides small but severe instances of poverty.[4] In the past it has been argued that mortality figures in rural areas suggest better healthcare outcomes, but people are now challenging this idea.[5]

Inequalities in health outcomes

Mortality for road traffic accidents,[6,7] asthma[8] and cancer[9] is worse in rural areas. Cancer is diagnosed at a later stage[10] and intervention rates for coronary artery disease lower.[11] Rural patients are admitted to hospital less frequently than urban patients.[12] Screening interventions for mammography and diabetic retinopathy reduce with distance. A combination of absolute health deprivation (the absence of services or a delay or physical barrier to provision of medical services) and socioeconomic deprivation can lead to quite distressing individual experiences of health care.

Socioeconomic inequalities in rural areas

··

Case scenario 1

A patient with bronchial carcinoma has developed bony metastases, confirmed by X-ray at the local hospital. Discussion with palliative care and with the oncologist confirms radiotherapy as the treatment of choice for pain relief. The patient states that he wishes to die at home, near to friends and family, not at a hospital 75 miles away. He adamantly refuses admission: his family and friends cannot afford the cost of travel to see him and the pain is such that he cannot consider two hours in an ambulance.

The relationship between socioeconomic deprivation and health is well established. Traditionally, rural areas have been regarded as relatively free from poverty. Increasingly however it is recognised that this is due to a failure of deprivation markers to identify small pockets of deprivation in otherwise affluent communities; using markers that are inappropriate; and even excluding small communities from analysis. This has led to the description of 'ecological fallacy' where the needs of a relatively small disadvantaged sector of a community are ignored because a statistical analysis reveals low levels of deprivation. Rural communities are particularly prone to a failure of the current analytical tools. The relationship between deprivation and health is just as important in rural areas. It is reported that:

> health is equally dependent on socio-economic status in urban wards and comparable rural areas. The large apparent urban–rural gradient in the relationship at ward level was a statistical artefact produced by an inconsistent scale of analysis and the geographical distribution of rich and poor. In the UK, large districts of similar housing types in cities and towns tend to concentrate people with similar socio-economic characteristics, while in rural areas not even small enumeration districts contain homogeneous populations. ... While average deprivation scores for a ward may give a reliable impression of the relative level of 'need' in an urban environment, they are misleading in a rural context.[13]

In Scotland health inequalities between those living in affluent and deprived areas are increasing over time. Increases have been particularly great in remote rural areas and especially among the rural elderly, probably due to growing socioeconomic inequalities among this group.[14]

Absolute health deprivation

In rural areas, independent of socioeconomic circumstances, health services cannot be guaranteed to the same level as in urban areas. This can be unavoidable due to a condition where the outcome is heavily dependent on time to access definitive care. Deficiencies may also be due to economic factors, such as the expense of providing ambulances, or the need to access highly specialised services such as angioplasty or trauma care that need to be situated where the appropriate skills can be concentrated most effectively. Rural primary care health teams have an obligation to develop and sustain appropriate clinical pathways, or develop local services to mitigate the disadvantages of poor access. Tension often exists between specialists who fail to recognise the need to compromise on what they perceive as quality, and primary care professionals who see that effective care is unobtainable for large sectors of their community.

Emergencies and acute care

....

Case scenario 2

You receive a phone call from a patient saying that he is at the roadside next to a badly damaged vehicle. A 999 response has been requested from the ambulance. A few minutes later, ambulance control requests your attendance; the local ambulance is not in the station, and is returning from the district general hospital 75 miles away. Its estimated time of arrival is 45 minutes.

....

Certain popular assumptions about acute health care are challenged in rural areas. For example, there are clear national targets that apply to emergency ambulance response times. These are less stringent for rural areas, but even then, for a fairly remote area or when the ambulance is not in the station, an emergency response within the appropriate timeframe cannot be achieved. Under these circumstances the GP is likely to be expected to respond by his or her community, but also because of his or her duties as a doctor.[15] Such circumstances may include a collapse in the community, road traffic accidents, maternity care or indeed any acute medical emergency perceived or real. Interventions by GPs can be very effective.[16]

GP involvement with medical emergencies can improve outcomes. Thrombolysis of myocardial infarction was reported in a GP community hospital before being available in many district general hospitals and rural GPs led the use of thrombolysis in a community setting,[17,18] which is now well established. Challenges for the future include rapid access to angioplasty and thrombolysis for stroke. A GP-led community hospital in Galloway already delivers thrombolysis for stroke.

Management of chronic conditions

Because of distance from community, family and friends, patients often choose to be managed at home rather than in hospital. This is particularly true for palliative care, but also for many other chronic conditions. As well as providing what is generally regarded as secondary care, rural GPs are much less likely to be supported effectively by specialist outreach services. As a result, the burden of clinical care lies with the primary care team. Repeated journeys to specialist centres, regularly up to 300 miles round-trip, mean individuals must travel thousands of miles for admissions and appointments.[19] Urban patients are three times more likely to receive some form of specialist care than those living more than three hours' travel from a regional centre, although a significant reduction in accessing specialist care exists for those travelling more than one hour.[20] It is reasonable to presume that these are causally related. It can be extrapolated from this that patients are either not receiving any care, or are receiving care from their GP through a health centre or community hospital.

For haemodialysis,[21,22] in response to evidence that travelling times in excess of 37 minutes had an impact on take-up rates (and presumably survival), Scotland has developed national guidelines. The provision of satellite units has improved take-up rates considerably. This simple addition to a guideline transforms the lives of many yet has little additional effect on primary care.

GP management of conditions that are usually managed in secondary care affects all socioeconomic groups. The cost of travel, both financial and time, will be a factor that will disproportionately affect the poor, elderly and infirm. In responding to this, there will be primary care workload issues both in consultation time and maintaining adequate quality of service. In summary patients often fail to access secondary care because of the need to travel. If we wish to deal with this inequality, we need to deliver secondary care locally through a combination of community hospitals, satellite units and enabling primary care to respond. Failing that, rural patients will continue to suffer unnecessarily from inequities in the delivery of health care.

Unscheduled care

One of the most fundamental changes to general practice has been the loss of 24-hour responsibility for general practice. This has been replaced by a much more centralised form of service delivery, using call centres that often do not have local knowledge, and GP cooperatives and primary care centres, often some distance from the patient. Patients in rural areas are less likely to contact the call centre.[23] This was unexpected, as seeking telephone advice should be equally accessible to all groups. This study also noted the compounding effect of deprivation in rural patients. Following a call, patients are also less likely to be seen by a GP directly related to the distance from a call centre.[24]

The development of a national nurse-led triage service and telephone advice should have improved the quality of service, and should certainly have reduced inequities. Evidence from Scotland suggests this has not happened;[25] a Medline search could not find any analysis of the telephone triage service, NHS Direct, on rural areas.

Holistic care in rural practice

Life as a GP in a rural area is often described as 'like living in a goldfish bowl'. Over time, most doctors will develop an intimate relationship with a community, which they serve, and are rewarded with personal and professional respect. Being aware of the personal and social circumstances of patients is the norm rather than the exception. For most patients, the doctor quickly becomes aware of the social, family and occupational circumstances of the individual. This personal information about knowledge, beliefs and expectations encourages a more dynamic advocacy role for individuals who wish to diverge from the more didactic approach encouraged by current guidelines and targets. Conversely, the doctor has to be careful that his or her personal knowledge of the patient does not conflict with offering and encouraging the best possible evidence-based treatment; there is a risk that knowledge of the social determinants of health can lead to ignoring or making judgements about physical health problems. For patients with chaotic lifestyles, these will all be well known to the primary care health team; even new patients will quickly be identified, and in a small practice it is much easier to develop a consistent approach while remaining accessible. When such patients cause difficulties or dilemmas for the practice, this personal knowledge can be used to support other professionals.

Solutions that have been proposed

Telehealth

It has been suggested that telehealth and telemedicine can deliver better outcomes for remote patients. A Cochrane report on electronic medical records (including patient records, clinical administration systems, digital imaging and archiving systems, e-prescribing, e-booking), telemedicine and telecare services, health information networks, decision support tools for healthcare professionals, and internet-based technologies and services found only nine randomised controlled trials. The search generated a total of 47,979 references and selected 63 studies for detailed evaluation. The authors' conclusion was:

Given the scarcity of available research in the field of ICT [information and communications technology] implementation, there is an urgent need to develop a knowledge base to support the design, implementation and evaluation of interventions aimed at promoting the optimal integration of ICT in all groups of healthcare professionals' practice.[26]

It is difficult at this moment in time to promote telemedicine over traditional proven methodology. Moreover technical issues, including bandwidth availability, mobile 3 and 4G cover and even frequent power supply problems, may limit its availability. The picture archiving and communication system (PACS), a centralised radiology database, allows images to be assessed remotely and is invaluable in obtaining telephone advice.

Outreach services

Specialist outreach services have been shown to benefit patients and GPs.[27] Helicopters have a role to play in delivering specialist support to medical, surgical and anaesthetic emergencies. Evidence of helicopter transfer improving clinical outcome is hard to find, and they may be unavailable for service reasons or bad weather or darkness. These do not replace the requirement to apply resuscitation skills for the first hour or even few hours of any acute illness. Remote decision support is the term used for contacting a consultant or other colleague who has knowledge and experience of the condition that is being managed, and who can give appropriate advice with regard to the clinical problem and the appropriate response for a rural setting. The rural GP should be able to develop a network to facilitate decision-making in a particular practice setting.

Community hospitals

Alongside the proposals to develop polyclinics in urban England, there was also support for community hospitals.[28] It is not clear whether these hospitals will be positioned in such a way that they will improve services for rural areas. Failure to do this risks duplicating urban services, at the same time reducing access to hospital care for rural areas. In England, the government assesses the performance of rural hospitals with the same criteria of cost and effectiveness that are applied to urban hospitals. No concession is made to compensating for geographically inaccessible services, or to diseconomies of scale.

Community hospitals provide better access to services for patients, and this should improve service uptake. The challenge is also to provide a quality of service that equals or exceeds that elsewhere. There is a cost for that, both in terms of diseconomies of scale and also the need for staffing at a senior level. The way forward appears to be to develop a generalist who can provide clinical care of an extended nature within a hospital setting. This will require specific training, and will present challenges with validation and accreditation.

What do rural and remote GPs need to know? Empowering rural primary care

This will vary from area to area, even between practices. What is certain is that a wider range of knowledge and skills is required, as is a personal ability to be flexible and improvise. Many of the skills and abilities that are required may only be called upon a few times in any one career. There is no area of expertise in which a rural GP should have a minimal competency that is less than an urban GP; however, depending on where he or she is situated and the nature of services expected, many additional skills might be expected from a rural GP. Depending on personal skills and experience these may not be available, resulting in a patient experiencing a different type of care.

RCGP Scotland examined the core competencies of a GP,[29] and made some additions. While the generality, the essential features of the discipline of everyone entering general practice, were not added to, a number of specific areas were augmented to reflect the needs of the rural or remote GP.

These additional training needs can be divided into two main areas: clinical competencies and personal qualities.

Clinical competencies

Looking at what rural GPs themselves think are the core values of their own practice (see Table 11.1), distance from a general hospital and dealing with minor injuries are most commonly regarded as defining rural practice. Both require the ability to provide services that would lie outside primary care for urban practices. Many of the generic skills required for this extended role in general practice are transferable across various disciplines; for example, basic life support is applied according to internationally agreed guidelines that are taught in a number of courses. They can be obtained by attending 'firedrill' type courses, which are often internationally recognised.

Table 11.1 **Reasons why GPs consider themselves rural**

	Percentage	Number
Distance from district general hospital	79.6%	109
Minor injury services	62.8%	86
Distance from nearest town	56.9%	78
Dispensing	55.5%	76
Distance from neighbouring practice	52.6%	72
Pre-hospital care	47.4%	65
Island	24.1%	33
Hospital work	24.1%	33
Single handed	16.1%	22
Maternity care	14.6%	20

Source: from a survey done by the RCGP Rural Practice Standing Group.

Pre-hospital care is a very important issue because ambulance response times can be poor, transfer times greater and either by design or default the GP will become involved. Many courses exist to develop these skills, such as the internationally transferable qualifications ATLS, ALS, PALS and ALSO. The British Association for Immediate Care Schemes (BASICS), which has both an English and a Scottish BASICs (see Table 11.2, overleaf), runs excellent courses and even has a diploma for the most enthusiastic.[30,31] Other examples of this might be suturing, minor injuries and follow-up of fractures or medical conditions that would normally be dealt with within a secondary care setting. This results in care that is quite different from urban areas, sometimes better, sometimes not. If we fail to address the latter, then health inequalities will increase.

Personal qualities

It would be wrong to suggest that rural GPs are inherently any better or worse than any other doctor. Practising medicine in a rural area creates a mixture of responsibilities and privileges that is rapidly disappearing in mainstream general practice. Being part of a community creates difficulty with confidentiality (both patient confidentiality and the privacy of the doctor and his or her family). The need to treat friends and sometimes even family creates pressures within the consultation. When things go wrong, the effects are far more likely to cross the divide between profes-

Table 11.2 **BASICS courses**

BASICS UK	BASICS Scotland
Pre-Hospital Care Course (PhEC)	Immediate Medical Care Course – Part 1 (IMC – Part 1)
Advanced PhEC	Immediate Medical Care Course – Part 2 (IMC – Part 2)
Five-day course	Immediate Medical Care Refresher Course (IMCR)
Refresher Course	Pre-Hospital Paediatric Life Support Course (PHPLS)
Pre-Hospital Paediatric Life Support Course (PhPLS)	Pre-Hospital Emergency Care Course (PHECC)
Paediatric Education for Pre-Hospital Professionals (PEPP)	Emergency Medicine Course (EMC)
Smart @ Scene	Pre-Hospital Paediatric Life Support (PHPLS)
	Major Incident Medical Management & Support Course (MIMMS)

sional and personal responsibility, whether as a result of error or not. This can lead to conflict and personal distress. The doctor must develop coping strategies and support networks that suit the practice demography.

Summary

From the evidence presented thus far, it might be argued that making central services more accessible to patients is the way forward for healthcare policy, for example having large polyclinics or community hospitals with better transport links. Distance from the GP surgery, rather than from hospital, is associated with an increased risk of emergency admissions, and a lower rate of other admissions for in-patient management.[32] Survival from cancer is related to travel time to the GP. When travel time to the hospital and other accessibility measures were taken into account, the travel to the GP was found to be the only influential factor.[33]

Looking at other values of general practice within rural communities, the concept of social capital is important. Social capital is the importance of certain organisations or infrastructures within a community. Examples of this might be school, church and medical practice. It is a very ill-defined concept, but is easily recognised within a rural community. However difficult it is to define or measure, it is an important concept and remains a key part of rural general practice.[34] This sense of community and cohesion is difficult to find in a modern urban society. It was once the essence of all general practice, and has been replaced by a restless, selfish and unsettled society. Mainstream general practice has been led unwittingly or otherwise along the same path. It may be helpful for managers and politicians to reinvigorate the concept of health services as social capital rather than commodity; although unfashionable, such an attitude still exists throughout the NHS and in a very holistic way benefits patients, society and professionals.

....

Applied Knowledge Test (AKT) questions

....

1 Which is a likely characteristic that defines practice as rural?

a Distance from neighbouring practice

b Hospital work

c Distance from district general hospital

d List size

e Single-handed

....

2 Which of the following statements is true about deprivation in rural areas?

a Deprivation is not a problem in rural areas

b Deprivation scores accurately reflect the situation in rural areas

c There is an effective tool for measuring rural deprivation

d Car ownership is an accurate reflection of rural socioeconomic deprivation

e Socioeconomic deprivation affects health for rural populations

....

Answers: **1 = a, c | 2 = e**

Acknowledgement: Dr David Hogg, Arran Medical Group, Isle of Arran, Scotland.

....

References

1. Farmer J C, Baird A G, Iversen L. Rural deprivation: reflecting reality. *British Journal of General Practice* 2001; **51 (467)**: 486–91.

2. Cox J. Rural general practice. *British Journal of General Practice* 1994; **44 (386)**: 388–9.

3. Asthana S, Gibson A. Rationing in response to NHS deficits: rural patients are likely to be affected most. *British Medical Journal* 2005; **331(7530)**: 1472.

4. Cox J. Poverty in rural areas. *British Medical Journal* 1998; **316(7133)**: 722.

5. Gartner A, Farewell D, Dunstan F, *et al*. Differences in mortality between rural and urban areas in England and Wales, 2002–04. *Health Statistics Quarterly* 2008; **39**: 61–113.

6. Bentham G. Proximity to hospital and mortality from motor vehicle traffic accidents. *Social Science & Medicine* 1986; **23(10)**: 1021–6.

7. Miles-Doan R, Kelly S. Inequities in health care and survival after injury among pedestrians: explaining the urban/rural differential. *Journal of Rural Health* 1995; **11(3)**: 177–84.

8. Jones AP, Bentham G. Health service accessibility and deaths from asthma in 401 local authority districts in England and Wales, 1988–92. *Thorax* 1997; **52(3)**: 218–22.

9. Campbell NCE, Sharp AM, Ritchie L, *et al*. Rural factors and survival from cancer: analysis of Scottish cancer registrations. *British Journal of Cancer* 2000; **82(11)**: 1863–6.

10. Campbell NCE, Sharp AM, Ritchie L, *et al*. Rural and urban differences in stage at diagnosis of colorectal and lung cancers. *British Journal of Cancer* 2001; **84(7)**: 910–14.

11. Hippisley-Cox J, Pringle M. Inequalities in access to coronary angiography and revascularisation: the association of deprivation and location of primary care services. *British Journal of General Practice* 2000; **50(455)**: 449–54.

12. Haynes R, Bentham G, Lovett A, *et al*. Effects of distances to hospital and GP surgery on hospital inpatient episodes, controlling for needs and provision. *Social Science & Medicine* 1999; **49(3)**: 425–33.

13. Huff N, Macleod C, Ebdon D, *et al*. Inequalities in mortality and illness in Trent NHS Region. *Journal of Public Health Medicine* 1999; **21(1)**: 81–7.

14. Levin KA, Leyland AH. A comparison of health inequalities in urban and rural Scotland. *Social Science & Medicine* 2006; **62(6)**: 1457–64.

15. General Medical Council. *Good Medical Practice*. London: GMC, 2013, www.gmc-uk.org/guidance/good_medical_practice.asp [accessed August 2013].

16. Cox J, Chapman TG. General practitioner attendance at emergencies notified to ambulance control. *British Medical Journal Clinical Research* Ed 1984; **289(6438)**: 165–6.

17. Gordon I. Streptokinase used in general practice. *Journal of the Royal College of General Practitioners* 1989; **39(319)**: 49–51.

18. Rawles J, Sinclair C, Jennings K, *et al*. Audit of prehospital thrombolysis by general practitioners in peripheral practices in Grampian. *Heart* 1998; **80(3)**: 231–4.

19. Baird AG, Donnelly CM, Miscampell NT, *et al*. Centralisation of cancer services in rural areas has disadvantages. *British Medical Journal* 2000; **320(7236)**: 717.

20. Baird G, Flynn R, Baxter G, *et al*. Travel time and cancer care: an example of the inverse care law? *Rural & Remote Health* 2008; **8(4)**: 1003.

21. Brammah A, Young G, Allan A, *et al*. Haemodialysis in a rural area: a demanding form of treatment. *Health Bulletin* 2001; **59(5)**: 294–9.

22. Roderick P, Clements S, Stone N, *et al*. What determines geographical variation in rates of acceptance onto renal replacement therapy in England? *Journal of Health Services Research & Policy* 1999; **4(3)**: 139–46.

23. Turnbull J, Martin D, Lattimer V, *et al.* Does distance matter? Geographical variation in GP out-of-hours service use: an observational study. *British Journal of General Practice* 2008; **58(552)**: 471–7.

24. O'Reilly D, Stevenson M, McCay C, *et al.* General practice out-of-hours service, variations in use and equality in access to a doctor: a cross-sectional study. *British Journal of General Practice* 2001; **51(469)**: 625–9.

25. Roberts A, Heaney D, Haddow G, *et al.* Implementation of a national, nurse-led telephone health service in Scotland: assessing the consequences for remote and rural localities. *Rural & Remote Health* 2009; **9(2)**: 1079.

26. Gagnon M, Legare F, Labrecque M, *et al.* Interventions for promoting information and communication technologies adoption in healthcare professionals. In: *Cochrane Database of Systematic Reviews.* Issue 3. Chichester: Wiley, 2009.

27. Gruen RL, Weeramanthri TS, Knight SSE, *et al.* Specialist outreach clinics in primary care and rural hospital settings. Cochrane Effective Practice and Organisation of Care Group. *Cochrane Database of Systematic Reviews.* Issue 3. Chichester: Wiley, 2009.

28. Parliamentary business, 23 June 2009, www.publications.parliament.uk/pa/cm200809/cmhansrd/cm090623/text/90623w0028.htm   [accessed July 2013].

29. GP curriculum: overview, www.rcgp-curriculum.org.uk/extras/curriculum/index.aspx [accessed July 2013].

30. British Association for Immediate Care, www.basics.org.uk/.

31. BASICS Scotland, www.basics-scotland.org.uk/.

32. Haynes R, Bentham G, Lovett A, *et al.* Effects of distances to hospital and GP surgery on hospital inpatient episodes, controlling for needs and provision. *Social Science & Medicine* 1999; **49(3)**: 425–33.

33. Jones AP, Haynes R, Sauerzapf V, *et al.* Travel times to health care and survival from cancers in Northern England. *European Journal of Cancer* 2008; **44(2)**: 269–74.

34. Farmer J, Lauder W, Richards H, *et al.* Dr John has gone: assessing health professionals' contribution to remote rural community sustainability in the UK. *Social Science & Medicine* 2003; **57(4)**: 673–86.

12 Intersectoral action as a strategy for primary health care to reduce health inequity

Sara Willems and Jan De Maeseneer

Aim

The aim of this chapter is to highlight the potential of intersectoral action (IA) as a strategy for primary health care to reduce inequity in health. The chapter describes in what contexts an IA approach provides added value over a single-sector (e.g. primary health care) approach and how IA can be adopted at several levels (global, national, community). It presents the underlying mechanisms and models for IA and describes community-oriented primary care (COPC) as a method to implement IA in the primary healthcare sector.

Key learning points

- Understand that the determinants of health are related to different sectors and that this is reflected in daily practice.

- Realise that there are boundaries in the physician's capacity to address the wider social determinants of a patient's health.

- Gain insight into how the IA for health approach can contribute to the reduction of health inequity.

- Understand for which goals an IA approach can be adopted and at what levels it can operate for health care.

- Appreciate that IA is guided by underlying theoretical models or frameworks and that the chosen model has implications for the actions to take.

- Understand how the COPC approach works and get insight into how it can be a useful method in addressing health inequity.

- Know the basic conditions or assumptions for successful IAs.

Primary health care: concept and features

In its most simple formulation, primary care is the first point of contact that people have with the health services.[1,2] IA for health is:

> essential health care based on practical, scientifically sound and socially acceptable methods and technology made univer-

sally accessible to individuals and families in the community through their full participation and at a cost that the community and the country can afford to maintain at every stage of their development in the spirit of self-reliance and self-determination.[3]

This ideal model of health care was adopted in the declaration of the International Conference on Primary Health Care held in Alma-Ata, Kazakhstan, in 1978 (known as the 'Alma-Ata Declaration'), and became a core concept of the World Health Organization's goal of 'Health for All'.[1,3]

In 1985 Vuori suggested that primary care should not only be seen as a set of activities, but also as a level of care, as a strategy for organising health care and as a philosophy that permeates health care.[4] Hereby Vuori stressed the importance of the paradigm shift from primary *medical* to primary *health* care. The central attributes of primary health care are: first contact (accessibility), continuity and longitudinality (personal-focused preventive and curative care over time) and patient-oriented comprehensiveness and coordination (including, when appropriate, referral towards secondary and tertiary care).[5] This means that the primary healthcare team deals with continuous care for all unselected health problems in all patient groups, irrespective of social class, religion, ethnicity, etc. The team deals with early signs and symptoms and combines person-centred cure, care and prevention. The emphasis is on effective and efficient diagnostic and therapeutic interventions. Continuity of care is essential and contributes to cost-effectiveness. Primary health care starts from the exploration of the needs and expectations of the patient and focuses on the empowering of individual health and strength (health promotion), addresses individual and cultural norms and values, and takes, when needed, the advocacy role. Moreover, a primary healthcare team acts as the hub in the navigation of the patient in the healthcare system.[1]

From patient to community: thinking outside the patient-level medical box

The case scenarios below illustrate the boundaries of the individual, patient-focused medical approach. They stimulate thinking outside the 'medical box' and shifting the focus from patients to the broader context of the community.

....

Case scenario 1: traffic safety

Three times in two months the team of the community health centre has to intervene urgently at the occasion of an accident where a schoolboy is hit by a car and seriously injured while crossing the street near the health centre. Every day, 500 schoolchildren have to cross that particular street and this is a dangerous situation. Instead of continuing to respond to emergencies, and calling ambulances to take the injured children to the hospital, the team decides to attack the root cause of the problem: the unsafe traffic situation in the neighbourhood. An action team is put in place, including representatives from the schools, youth organisations, organisations for elderly people, the police, etc. Also the neighbours are invited to participate. Together, this group succeeds in convincing the local policymakers to improve the traffic situation in the street and make it more safe for pedestrians. A concerted action plan is designed: the schools in the neighbourhood organise lessons on road safety, youth movements organise activities where children learn advanced biking skills. An evaluation after five years shows that there were no more traffic accidents with impaired pedestrians in the neighbourhood.

....

Case scenario 2: pregnant teenagers

Wendy, aged 17 years, is consulting: she became pregnant by a boy she met at a party some months ago. Although she is not in a relationship with this boy, she wants to keep the baby. Wendy is unemployed and was unsuccessful in her career as a student. In a first approach, the GP thinks Wendy became pregnant because she was not informed about contraception or didn't know how to use it appropriately, and he addresses the topic. But in the consultation it becomes clear that Wendy knows exactly how to use contraception. Two weeks later, Kelly, aged 16 years, presents with a similar story: she became pregnant, is not in a stable relationship, has no job, has had a difficult student career.

After two months, it becomes clear that there is a 'teenager pregnancy epidemic' in the neighbourhood.

The pregnant girls seem to know each other. In order to understand the background of those pregnancies, a focus group led by an anthropologist is organised to explore the motivation of the girls. The findings are that they made a deliberate choice to get pregnant, that the child is considered as an 'existential' sign of their fundamental right to procreation, and that it is their own decision. Professionals from the different sectors in the neighbourhood decide to work together and to organise the care for the girls and their babies, and to empower them as a team, but also to organise activities in the neighbourhood to prevent more girls becoming pregnant.

....

....

Case scenario 3: the Bromley-by-Bow Health Centre in London

Author: Dr Sam Everington, WONCA Europe Five-Star Doctor 2006

....

The Bromley-by-Bow Health Centre has developed over a number of years as a partnership between the public, private and voluntary sector and patients. It started as a church that was converted in 1984 into a health centre and which opened in 1997. The café and art wing opened in 2000 and the 'Enterprise Bar' in 2005. Its philosophy is integration of over 100 different projects, a sharing of all spaces and a living building that matches the functions of those working and using the centre. The centre is contracted by the local authority to manage the two-acre park it sits in, and it delivers a safe and beautiful space for the local community. The philosophy is to improve the health of the community you have, addressing not just traditional health issues, but also people's other health needs – employment, education, the environment and creativity. The centre is owned by the community and with a 'can do' culture supports all to manage and improve their health and to become 'social entrepreneurs'. The centre integrates all ages and cultural groups, and supports all in the community to be partners as much as users and actively participate. It backs people before structures. The local community is 50% Bengali and 25% other ethnic minority groups. At least a third of the community uses the centre on a regular basis and 90% at least once a year. The users of the centre completely reflect the demography of the area.

....

Towards intersectoral action for health

History

The concept of IA was also introduced at the International Conference on Primary Health Care in Alma-Ata in 1978. The primary healthcare model adopted by the conference explicitly stated the need for 'a comprehensive health strategy that not only provides health services but also addresses the underlying social, economic and political causes of poor health'.[5,6] In the following years the need to work between sectors to realise health gains was further emphasised by international organisations and governments but little results in the field were reported. In the 1990s the knowledge on determinants of health increased importantly, so were the efforts to work across sectors to address them. The recent publication of several reports by the European Union and by the WHO, describing and analysing good practices in IA, reflects the increasing implementation of the concept on the global, national or local level.[5,7,8]

Definition and goals of intersectoral action

The definition of IA has been the subject of an extensive debate. At the one end of the spectrum, initiatives that simply share information or coordinate actions undertaken by different sectors are considered as IA. Towards the other end of the same spectrum, IA initiatives are intertwined with collaborative actions between sectors, with each sector inputting meaningful resources and expertise towards a shared analysis, coordinated intervention and common outcomes.

The definition formulated in 1997 by the WHO conference on Intersectoral Action for Health states that:

> Intersectoral Action for Health is a recognised relationship between a part of or parts of the health care sector with a part of or parts of another sector which has been formed to take action on an issue to achieve health outcomes (or intermediate health outcomes) in a way that is more effective, efficient or sustainable than could be achieved by the health sector acting alone.[9]

An example of this in the new UK NHS commissioning landscape would be Joint Strategic Needs Assessments (JSNAs), which are developed with the involvement of local public health agencies, council representatives, education and police as well as primary care.

IA is a strategy that can address a wide range of health problems and socioeconomic public policy challenges. In general, three categories of key goals of IA for health can be identified.[5,8]

First, an IA approach can be adopted to *enhance health outcomes across the population*.

....

For instance projects to increase the knowledge of adolescents about STDs in which the health sector collaborates with the educational sector (e.g. schools) and the entertainment sector (e.g. TV programmes for adolescents) to reach the target group.

....

These initiatives may or may not contribute to a reduction in the inequity gap between social classes and, if they do, this is not the primary focus. Interventions with this goal might have a geographical focus, e.g. underserved or rural areas, but the actions focus on the whole population in these areas, not on specific categorical subgroups.

Second, an IA approach can be adopted to address the *determinants of health*.

The implementation of a series of five-year economic plans has resulted in improvements in literacy, female employment rates, nutrition and sanitation in Malaysia. These improvements also had a positive impact on the health of the nation.

Health improvements might be considered as one potential benefit of these interventions but they are not identified as the primary objective.

Third, IA initiatives can also explicitly aim at *reducing health inequity* between specified groups. They involve programmes that are targeted at a population of interest or use a combination of selective and universal approaches (so called 'proportionate universalism').

The UK government set a national target to narrow the gap in life expectancy by area and the infant mortality by social class. Hereto a comprehensive national strategy was developed to support the targets which included actions and interventions on smoking, housing quality, injuries, diet, immunization and poverty reduction. Intersectoral action was hereby indentified as a critical requirement and both universal (e.g. improving accessibility of care) and selective approaches (e.g. initiatives focusing on the poorest population groups) were initiated.

Although the value of IA for health is widely recognised, it cannot be considered as superior to single-sector action for health. The question of which approach is appropriate given a set of circumstances does not lead to a straightforward answer. An important factor for consideration is the degree of control or influence over an intended target or outcome. If a single sector exercises complete or near-complete control over an issue, single-sectoral action may be appropriate. When multiple sectors share control over an issue, or when a sector wishes to influence a target over which it has less control, IA may be more appropriate. Other determining factors for the choice between IA and single-sector action may include previous experience with bringing diverse sectors together, the existence of supporting (policy) structures and the level of trust between the partners.[8]

Intersectoral action for health at different levels of decision-making

Health and health inequity are determined by a large number of interrelating factors acting at different levels: at the micro-level of the individual patient, e.g. lifestyle and health-related behaviour; at the nano-level of the immediate social context, e.g. health beliefs of friends and family members; at the community level (meso-level), e.g. traffic safety in the neighbourhood; and at the macro-level, e.g. the organisation of the national health (care) system or – the scarce – European health regulations.[10] Parallel with the multi-level origin of social inequity, interventions to tackle inequity should be taken at all levels of decision-making: at global, national and local level. At all levels intersectoral approaches can be adopted to set up effective interventions.[5]

At the *global level* the WHO and other United Nations agencies are regular initiators of IA for health initiatives.[5]

In the 'Health for All' declaration of 1978 the WHO stated that it should focus primarily on attaining by the year 2000 a level of health that enables all individuals to lead a socially and economically productive life. In the following decades this intention was renewed in several declarations. Health for All became the global health policy framework of WHO that forms the basis of a global movement and a driver of the action in the member states.[11]

Another interesting initiative at the regional level was undertaken by the European Union, which adopted health impact assessments (HIAs) as a tool to identify linkages between health and other sectoral policies.[8] It is a combination of methods whose aim is to assess the health consequences to a population of a policy, project or programme that does not necessarily have health as its primary objective.[12, 13]

At *national level*, many countries have used intersectoral approaches to address complex, multifaceted issues, combining the efforts of the relevant government departments and societal agencies into a single coordinated strategy.

In a recent report the Public Health Agency of Canada provided an overview of IA approaches, with the national policies of the UK and Sweden being described as examples of nationwide IA initiatives. In these countries broad policy frameworks or whole-of-government approaches are adopted to address the social gradient in health.[5]

A critical factor in national-level initiatives is the complexity of the government structure. This complexity is defined in terms of the number of levels of government as well as the distribution of legislative responsibilities across the levels. The implementation of national-level IA initiatives seems to be easier in government structures where the division of responsibilities concerning health or key determinants of health is transparent and simple. When this is not the case, the implementation of IA is much more complex and challenging.[8]

> In Belgium different levels of government bear different responsibilities for health and social determinants of health: curative health care services are a federal responsibility, public health services including prevention and health promotion are a regional responsibility – as are education and social housing – and the responsibility for income assistance is located at different levels depending on the type of assistance. IAs designed to reduce inequities are therefore difficult to implement on a national level and the actions that have been implemented in Belgium focus mainly on regional and local levels.[8]

In an analysis of 18 country case studies, performed by the WHO and the Public Health Agency of Canada, it is speculated that whole-of-government approaches that originate at the national level are limited in their capacity to influence some of the key social determinants of health if such initiatives are not supported by comprehensive, bottom-up initiatives that occur at the national levels. The report illustrates this with the example of the UK, where a strong horizontal integration of sectors at national level was accompanied by a weaker vertical integration with the local level and with inconsistent IA at this local level. This appeared to limit the impact of the overall, nationwide strategy.[8]

At the *community or local level*, IA often brings together a wide range of actors such as clinicians, social workers, researchers, local policymakers, civil society members (neighbourhood representatives, self-help groups, parent groups, etc.) and private sector actors (shop owners in the neighbourhood, producers of 'healthy goods', etc.) to collaborate to address areas of mutual interest.[5]

> In 2004 family physicians and school nurses working in deprived areas in Ghent (Belgium) noticed the high number of toddlers with bad dental health, permanently sucking a bottle with sweetened drinks. An intersectoral network of professionals was established: family physicians, community nurses, school workers, child and family health service workers, dentists, city council workers, researchers from the nearby university campus, etc., and an intersectoral action plan was designed (the Healthy Teeth Programme). First, the researchers set up a systematic screening in Ghent which revealed that 18% of children under the age of

30 months already had symptoms of caries, with higher rates in children living in the most deprived areas and in children with Eastern European mothers. None of the children with caries was ever treated. Inappropriate brushing behavior and bad feeding habits were identified as determinants of the early childhood caries. A qualitative study was set up, which showed the determinants of the dental health-related behavior of the parents. Lack of knowledge, barriers in the accessibility of the healthcare system and the difficulty in adopting appropriate parenting skills seemed to be important factors. An intersectoral intervention was set in place: educational materials on dental health were developed and used in local schools; local shop owners highlighted the availability of childrens' toothbrushes and toothpaste in their shops; agreements on accessibility of care with dentists in the neighborhood were made; all professionals working in the neighborhood received a manual with practical information about children's oral health (e.g. how frequently to brush a child's teeth); oral health was included as a point of attention in the child and family clinics; a parenting skills course was offered by the Centre for Parenting (e.g. how to say 'no' to a child who requests a bottle of soft drink at night); March became 'the month of teeth' during which the topic of healthy teeth was focused on in schools and community health centres.[14]

Many of these community-level initiatives facilitate active public participation and/or invite the local community to define problems and develop strategies to approach inequities in that area or neighbourhood.

Also the municipal government can play a very important role in community-level IA initiatives.

In the Healthy Teeth Programme the municipal government guaranteed the sustainability of the programme, years even after its initial start. The Department of Health of the City of Ghent established a 'resources library' where all the developed educational materials are kept up to date and where organisations can borrow them when needed for their activities. The City also regularly organises meetings with all the initial participants to keep them informed and organises new activities to keep the issue of dental health on the agenda. Over the years, this group became a standing working partner of the City Health Council, established in 2010.

Community-level initiatives can take up an extremely important role in tackling inequity in health. First, when there is no or little national commitment for addressing social determinants of health, effective initiatives can still be developed at a local level, especially if there is strong local support and a willingness to build community empowerment. The lack of a broad-based national strategy doesn't necessarily hamper the implementation of local strategies. Second, local-level work is vital to reduce social inequities even when there is a national-level commitment. Decentralisation is needed to incorporate the local context adequately in the strategies and to increase ownership by the local community. By doing so, chances of success are increased.[5,8]

Intersectoral action approaches

Intersectoral approaches can also be adopted at the level of the individual patient. A classic example is the situation of an undocumented migrant who consults with an anxiety disorder. In a first approach the 'upstream causes' of the anxiety will be explored: the fear of being expelled from the country; the difficulty of finding work; language and cultural barriers; and the lack of social cohesion in the neighbourhood the person is living in. An accessible interdisciplinary primary care health team will be able to address the various dimensions of the patient's problem: the physician will look at the anxiety disorder; the social worker will deal with the immigration status; a referral to an employment agency will help with finding an appropriate occupation; the adult education sector will contribute to learning the local language; and the community workers will plan activities to contribute to the integration of migrant populations and strengthening social cohesion. Very often, an intersectoral approach, also at the individual level, will be key in order to address problematic living conditions.

The need for a multilevel approach

Horizontal collaboration occurs when initiatives are taken across sectors or across sub-sectors within one sector, involving individuals or groups from the same political decision-level. Vertical collaboration is working across levels of decision-making or jurisdiction in order to address issues that require decisions by more than one level of government, e.g. national governments working with regional and local governments. The 2007 literature review[8] of the Public Health Agency of Canada stated that:

> intersectoral action is strongest, and outcomes are best, when the collaboration is both vertical and horizontal. ... [w]eaving these elements together yields a resilient and durable end product, and provides a shield against inaction, flagging interest, or disintegration. At the same time, because of the wide range of inter-

ests involved, additional effort and negotiation may be required to reach a shared understanding of goals, approaches, mutual roles, and accountability for outcomes.[5]

Key mechanisms and tools to support intersectoral action for health

An analysis of 18 country cases of IA identified a broad range of key mechanisms in the planning, implementation and evaluation of IA initiatives and several concrete tools. In this section we describe some of these key mechanisms and tools. The importance of each mechanism or applicability of a certain tool is not constant over all initiatives. Context determines to a large extent the success of the various mechanisms and tools. A specific context might enable significant policy action that in a different context or at a different time might be unsuccessful. Although the importance of the context is incontestable, there is no such thing as a single set of preconditions that are absolutely necessary to support IA. Yet, of some characteristics it can be said that they at least ease the development and implementation of strategies (e.g. existing networks between sectors). Also the lack of some factors (such as having centralised responsibilities concerning health and its determinants at the same level of jurisdiction) could be compensated by the more vigorous application of others (such as strong IA at the local level).[8]

Key to effective IA is the shared recognition among all protagonists that IA is a suitable strategy to address the common goal. Having a strong rationale for an intersectoral approach is absolutely necessary to get activities off the ground. 'Building the case for IA' can be achieved in several ways. Building on the public concern can be an effective way. The public expectation is – especially in large parts of Europe – generally one of social justice and equity. By 'feeding' this expectation, for instance by informing the public with new research data on inequity, the public concern about inequity might increase and so the pressure on the political agenda. Another way to build a case for IA is to use recognised leaders to advocate for IA. For national-level IA initiatives these can be political champions or senior government officials. At the community level family doctors, social workers, etc. can play this important role and stimulate the willingness of others to participate in an IA initiative. Other ways are to acknowledge the limitations of previous approaches (especially single-sector strategies), building consensus via shared gatherings such as conferences or community meetings, framing the issue in a way that all sectors could relate to, and building on high-profile international sponsorship, e.g. sponsorship by the United Nations or the European Union can be motivating, especially when there is no high-level commitment by national governments.[5,8]

Essential to IA is the collaboration of a variety of sectors. Setting up a process in which groups of people and organisations who do not know each other well have to share power and decision-making, is challenging. Building trust is a key issue when *engaging other sectors* in the development and maintenance of IA. Although this process is time-consuming and intensive, it's worthwhile since trust ensures a strong foundation for effective working relationships.

In the daily reality this process is frequently challenged by factors such as too many and varied mandates at the table, a high turnover of staff, cultural differences or different philosophies among the various partners, a history of poor working relationships that needs time to overcome, and bureaucratic regulations that make it difficult to share power across sectors.[8]

In a project to improve the accessibility of the Belgian healthcare system, the government established an intersectoral working group to formulate policy recommendations. This group consisted of the staff of several governmental departments, researchers, primary care workers, employers' organisations, organisations representing the poor, etc. It took several months to build a trusting working relationship between the participants. An important factor here was that the participating organisations for people living in poverty had experienced strong paternalism and 'fake' involvement in working groups and unrealistic expectations in the past. Also differences in the mandate of the representatives concerning decision-making, in the speed of progress, in style of meeting, etc. slowed the process of building trust.[8]

To overcome these challenges and strengthen these important relationships, it might be useful to communicate clearly about the type of collaboration expected from the different participants and to define what the collaboration exactly will look like. Moreover, once the process of partnership development has been established it can be useful to draw up formal agreements and memoranda of understanding between all parties.[5,8]

To organise IA for health a variety of *theoretical models or frameworks* can guide the action and many concrete *strategies, methods and tools* can be applied.

Due to the complexity of government roles and responsibilities, and the traditional silos often operating between national governmental departments, countries that adopt a national-level approach tend to develop formal models and frameworks to guide their IA.[5,8]

To guide their IA for health inequity, the government of New Zealand uses a theoretical framework that encourages planners to consider action at four different levels: the structural level (social, economic, cultural and historical factors that fundamentally determine health such as taxation and education), intermediary pathways (access to material resources, lifestyle, environment, etc.), health and disability services (access to care, health education, etc.), and the impact of disability and illness on socioeconomic position (income support, antidiscrimination legislation, etc.).[8]

With this formal model or framework as a theoretical guide, a common concrete way to organise actions at national level is the formation of inter-ministerial committees. These structures tend to lend credibility to the health (inequity) issue and to a cooperative approach. However, they can also create confusion and add unnecessary bureaucracy.[8]

The community level tends to require a more flexible and organic structure that can respond to community needs and preferences. In this context the COPC approach has been proven to be very useful.[8]

COPC as a method to support intersectoral action for health

COPC can be characterised as a primary healthcare approach that integrates individual and population-based care, blending the clinical skills of the practitioner with epidemiology, preventive medicine and health promotion. By doing so, it tries to minimise the separation between public health and individual health care, and to address the broader social determinants of health.[15] COPC has the community it works with as its most important patient. Here the 'community' can be predefined (e.g. all inhabitants of a village) or can be 'practice defined' (all patients in the practice).[16] The following highly desirable features are needed for a successful COPC approach:

- integration of curative and preventive care
- a comprehensible approach to behavioural, social and environmental determinants
- a multidisciplinary team and good relations with other community agencies
- a low threshold for community members to consult the team
- direct involvement of the community through its members.[17]

The COPC approach consists of an identification of the community, a systematic assessment of the health problems and healthcare needs in the community (a so-called 'community diagnosis'), the development and implementation of systematic interventions, and the monitoring of the impact of the interventions to ensure that the targets are met and the interventions are responsive to community needs.[18] Essential in the COPC approach is that community members are involved in every phase of the process and also in the selection of the goals. A team of primary care health workers and community members, preferably extended by professionals from other sectors, assesses resources and develops strategic plans to deal with the problems that have been identified.[19,20]

> A COPC exercise was implemented in Ledeberg, a deprived neighbourhood in Ghent, Belgium. The Community Health Center Botermarkt was confronted in the mid-1980s with a problem concerning the physical development of children. A survey revealed that children in the community spent two times longer in front of television and videogames than the Flemish average, and that the children took part in significantly less physical activity. Youth organisations, schools, parent organisations, etc. contributed to a community diagnosis: 'lack of playing ground for children'. As almost 10,000 people were living on 1 km², there was not much green space left. Therefore, extra playgrounds were constructed with the help of the city on one hand and of community volunteers on the other. Activities were organised during the holidays. An assessment demonstrated important outcomes: the police reported a decrease in street crime during the holidays, there was an increase in social cohesion as both the local Belgian community and children from the Turkish community participated in the activities, and there was an improvement in physical condition.

Over the years the implementation of the COPC model has encountered difficulties at several levels. The openness of national governments and the governmental priorities concerning health largely influence the public concern about community health problems and the climate for setting up COPC projects.[21]

Evolutions in the USA and in the UK show that different choices of the government, through financing, play an important role in the success of implementation of health care models such as COPC.[22]

Other obstacles to greater acceptance of the COPC model lie in traditional medical training that emphasises individual curative care, and the lack of epidemiological, social and behavioural skills of the physicians who follow this curriculum. However, the introduction of COPC models into the undergraduate medical curriculum has led to positive experiences.[10] Finally, the organisation of the healthcare and insurance systems in which primary care must work is of great importance. For example, a patient list per practice is not yet a common feature in all European countries, thus impairing the delineation of a target population in a COPC strategy.[16]

Monitoring the process and the outcomes of intersectoral action and ensuring sustainability

An essential phase in the development of interventions is the evaluation of the processes and outcomes. This is especially the case for IA since this approach is fairly recent and evidence for the overall effectiveness of the use of IA for health and health equity, and the applied tools, is not yet researched in depth.[8]

Evaluating IA is a rather difficult exercise. In national programmes, where objective measures are already available, it is difficult to ascribe improvements to the intersectoral activities or to continuation of longer-term trends in the national population. In local-level initiatives it would be easier to attribute improvements to the activities since it is easier to monitor the context in which the intervention takes place than at the national level. However, very often at this level systematic conclusions have not been formulated because no or insufficient data have been collected.[8] In this context inviting managers of health information systems as participants in the IA team might contribute to the evaluation process since these systems provide rich data on health and healthcare use.

In general, the experience of the current IA initiatives shows that IA becomes more difficult in more complex environments that have a high number of partners and interests, at global or national levels compared with local or community levels, or with many logistical challenges. However, more research is needed to strengthen this experience-based evidence.[5]

Reports on IA repeatedly show that intersectoral action for health tends to cost more and takes longer to achieve results than other approaches, which make it essential that all partners in the process make a long-term commitment. Yet sustaining intersectoral initiatives has been a challenge due to changes in government, emergency or public health crises shifting attention elsewhere, and/or staff turnover.[5]

IA is extremely resource-intensive in terms of people, money and time. However, the roles, actors, skills and resources needed are different in every phase of the IA process. For example, negotiation and resource-finding is crucial in the development stage and of less importance in the implementation or assessing-impact phase.[8] It is important that professionals in the various sectors are trained in the skills and knowledge needed to participate in IA teams. As family doctors often take up leadership and advocacy roles in IA, they should be prepared to take up these roles.

Conditions for effective intersectoral action: summary

In the above parts of this chapter various enabling factors and conditions for effective IA were presented. A comprehensive list of these conditions is provided in the report *Working Together: intersectoral action for health*. Box 12.1 acts as an easy-to-consult summary of this chapter and is included as help to the reader.[5,23]

Box 12.1 Conditions for effective IA

- The parties have identified a *need* to work together in order to achieve their goals. This requires clarity on individual organizational goals, as well as joint goals.

- In the broader operating environment, there are *opportunities* that promote intersectoral collaboration, e.g. the community understands and is supportive.

- Organizations and professionals have the *capacity* – the required resources, skills and knowledge – to take action.

- The parties have developed a *relationship* on which to base cooperative, planned action. The relationship is clearly defined and is based on trust and respect.

- The *planned action* is well conceived and can be implemented and evaluated. The action is clear and there is agreement to undertake it. Roles and responsibilities are clear.

- There are plans to *monitor* and *sustain outcomes from the start of the intervention*.

Source: adapted from Harris E, Wise M, Howe P. *Working Together: intersectoral action for health*.[23]

Applied Knowledge Test (AKT) questions

1   Which statement(s) is (are) not correct?

a   IA for health at local level is doomed to fail when there is no country-wide consensus or action plan on the topic

b   An IA approach that aims to increase literacy can also have an impact on the health of the population

c   Previous experience with IA for health is a precondition when setting up a new initiative

d   The participation of community members is essential in the COPC approach

2   Which of the following tools may contribute most to IA for health at community level?

a   The presence of an interdisciplinary primary care health centre

b   The use of evidence-based medical guidelines

c   The establishment of a platform where different sectors (police, housing, education, etc.) meet regularly

Answers: **1** = **a, c** | **2** = **c**

References

1. Starfield B. Is primary care essential? *Lancet* 1994; **344(8930)**: 1129–33.

2. De Maeseneer J, Willems S, De Sutter A, *et al.* Primary health care as a strategy for achieving equitable care: a literature review commissioned by the Health Systems Knowledge Network. 2007. www.who.int/social_determinants/resources/csdh_media/primary_health_care_2007_en.pdf   [accessed July 2013].

3. World Health Organization. *Declaration of Alma-Ata.* Adopted at the International Conference on Primary Health Care, Alma-Ata, USSR, 6–12 September 1978.

4. Vuori H. The role of the schools of public health in the development of primary health care. *Health Policy* 1985; **4(3)**: 221–30.

5. Public Health Agency of Canada. *Crossing Sectors: experiences in intersectoral action, public policy and health.* Ottawa, Ontario: PHAC, 2007, www.phac-aspc.gc.ca/publicat/2007/cro-sec/index-eng.php   [accessed August 2013].

6. WHO Commission on Social Determinants of Health. *Action on the Social Determinants of Health: learning from previous experiences.* Geneva: WHO Secretariat of the Commission on Social Determinants of Health, 2005, www.who.int/social_determinants/resources/action_sd.pdf   [accessed July 2013].

7. Stahl T, Wismar M, Ollila E, *et al. Health in All Policies: prospects and potentials.* Helsinki: Ministry of Social Affairs and Health, Health Department, Finland & European Observatory on Health Systems and Policies, 2006.

8. Public Health Agency of Canada, World Health Organization. *Health Equity through Intersectoral Action: an analysis of 18 country case studies.* Geneva: WHO, 2008, www.who.int/social_determinants/resources/health_equity_isa_2008_en.pdf   [accessed July 2013].

9. World Health Organization. *Intersectoral Action for Health: a cornerstone for health-for-all in the twenty-first century. Report to the International Conference 20–23 April 1997 Halifax, Nova Scotia, Canada.* Geneva: WHO, 1997.

10. Art B, De Roo L, Willems S, *et al.* An interdisciplinary community diagnosis experience in an undergraduate medical curriculum: development at Ghent University. *Academic Medicine* 2008; **83(7)**: 1040–6.

11. World Health Organization Europe. *The Health for All Policy Framework for the WHO European Region: 2005 update.* Copenhagen: WHO Regional Office for Europe, 2005, www.euro.who.int/en/publications/abstracts/health-for-all-policy-framework-for-the-who-european-region-the-2005-update   [accessed October 2013].

12. Scott Samuel A. Assessing how public policy impacts on health. *Healthlines* 1997; **47**: 15–17.

13. Kark S. *The Practice of Community-Oriented Primary Health Care.* New York: Appleton-Century-Crofts, 1981.

14. Willems S, Vanobbergen J, Martens L, *et al.* The independent impact of household- and neighborhood-based social determinants on early childhood caries: a cross-sectional study of inner-city children. *Family and Community Health* 2005; **28(2)**: 168–75.

15. Van Weel C, De Maeseneer J, Roberts R. Integration of personal and community health care. *Lancet* 2008; **362(9392)**: 1314–19.

16. De Maeseneer J, De Roo L, Art B, *et al.* Intersectoral action for health in Belgium: a multi-level contribution to equity. Internal document to the Knowledge Network 'Health Systems' of the Commission on Social Determinants of Health of WHO. www.who.int/social_determinants/resources/isa_multilevel_contribution_bel.pdf   [accessed July 2013].

17. Swanson R, Mosley H, Sanders D, *et al.* Call for global health-systems impact assessments. *Lancet* 2009; **374(9688)**: 433–5.

18. Rhyne R, Bogue R, Kukulka G, *et al. Community-Oriented Primary Care: health care for the 21st century.* Washington, DC: American Association for Public Health, 1998.

19. Koperski M, Rodnick J. Recent developments in primary care in the United Kingdom: from competition to community-oriented primary care. *Journal of Family Practice* 1999; **48(2)**: 140–5.

20. Epstein L, Gofin J, Gofin R, *et al.* The Jerusalem experience: three decades of service, research, and training in community-oriented primary care. *American Journal of Public Health* 2002; **92(11)**: 1717–21.

21. Tollman S. Community-oriented primary care: origins, evolution, applications. *Social Science & Medicine* 1991; **3296**: 633–42.

22. Whitehead M, Dahlgren G. *Concepts and Principles for Tackling Inequalities in Health: levelling up part 1*. Copenhagen: WHO, 2006.

23. Harris E, Wise M, Howe P. *Working Together: intersectoral action for health*. Canberra: Government Publishing Service, 1995.

13

The future of general practice
Challenges and opportunities

Gilles de Wildt and Paramjit Gill

Key learning points

- Have an awareness of external influences on the nature of general practice including commercialisation.

- Discuss the ethical implications of the challenges to general practice.

- Describe individual and collective responses to help protect vulnerable patients.

Introduction

What does the future hold for general practice in the UK? Which organisational and ethical challenges are GPs, GP registrars and other members of primary care teams likely to meet during, and beyond, the consultation?

Core issues are pay for performance, commercialisation, the increasing use of health information and challenges for maintaining long-term personal continuity of care. Central is the question: What can GPs do to protect professionalism and to help safeguard the position of the most vulnerable patients?

The government is the central actor in this field, interacting with other players in the health policy arena.[1] The latter include GPs, their professional organisations such as the Royal College of General Practitioners (RCGP) and the British Medical Association (BMA), larger and smaller for-profit and non-profit healthcare organisations, as well as patients' groups.

UK-wide pay for performance

In 2004, pay for performance was introduced in UK general practice through the Quality and Outcomes Framework (QOF),[2] linking the achievement of targets for a number of indicators to monetary rewards. Scores are publicly available, and make GP practices much more transparent, comparable and accountable. Doran and colleagues[3] found that, in the early stage, the QOF reduced inequalities as expressed in the scores for incentivised care in practices in deprived areas that had relatively poor performance before the QOF, while improvement in other practices levelled off. However, the King's Fund concluded three years later that over a longer period there was no evidence that the QOF either improved health or reduced inequalities.[4] Practices in deprived areas, however, need to work harder or require more health professionals and staff to 'get the points', thus worsening inequalities in terms of resourcing.

Roland[5] observed that quality was already improving with little or no monetary incentivisation, but improved further after 2004. He warned that the unmeasured, or not easily measurable, may lose importance and noted that 'external incentives are most likely to strengthen internal motivation where they support existing professional values, and may damage it when they don't'. He further suggested that GPs should now protect and improve the caring, interpersonal aspects of general practice. Heath and colleagues[6] warned that pay for performance on disease-specific targets can undermine the integrating, coordinating and very personal role of the GP. They also observed that most evidence is derived from studies in patients with single diseases, and not with co-morbidities, leaving much of the story of general practice untold.

Research in California-based primary care doctors reported resentment and a reduced sense of ownership under pay for performance arrangements, a phenomenon that was less present in UK GPs.[7] Furthermore, unexpectedly high QOF scores sharply raised GP partner incomes. In 2006, they earned 4.2 times the average income in the UK, occupying the top position among 21 Organisation for Economic Co-operation and Development (OECD) countries, above Mexico and the US.[8] This, combined with the withdrawal of the basic practice allowance per GP partner, led many partnerships to seek cheaper salaried doctors to fill vacancies, creating hierarchies and causing feelings of disenchantment and disillusion amongst non-principal GPs.[9]

Two further observations can be made. Kramer[10] and Scandinavian researchers[11] questioned the ethical justification for opportunistic prevention, which is central to the QOF, without offering an informed choice. It involves risk profiling, in future perhaps also on the basis of genetic testing. This may lead to discrimination and not do justice to the autonomy of patients, who may not wish to be screened for conditions for which they did not see the doctor. Indeed, in a qualitative study[12] most patients were unaware and surprised to hear about the QOF and that their practice was paid for 'simple things'.

Second, data collection systems can also be used for cost-control and commercial purposes. This is a particular challenge in England, where the government promotes the introduction of a market and brings in large for-profit corporations and other providers. In May 2013 it was reported that, after an approval process, companies can buy hospital data sets for £8000, including £140 to make records identifiable.[13]

Commercialisation: England goes a separate way

Scotland and Wales, with their internal autonomy over health, have chosen to block further commercialisation, fearing higher costs, reduced transparency and less cooperation within the service. While being confronted with the need for cost cutting, they maintain an essentially state-run integrated health service along traditional NHS lines.

This marks a stark contrast with England, where changes were heralded by events in July 2006. In order to comply with European competition law, the government placed an advert in the *Official Journal of the European Union*, inviting companies to express an interest in running budgets of Primary Care Trusts (PCTs) of the NHS. According to the *British Medical Journal*,[14] this raised 'the spectre of giant US healthcare firms being handed the bulk of the health service's £80bn budget'. When discovered, the advert 'united doctors, MPs, and campaign groups in fury against the government, which they accused of "privatisation by stealth"'. There had been no public or parliamentary announcement of the plans. The Secretary for Health apologised, stated that there was 'no question' of privatising the NHS, and withdrew the advert as it contained 'drafting errors'. Soon after, the advert was rewritten and placed again.

Earlier, the UK government ended the monopoly of provision of general practice by General Medical Services (GMS) or Personal Medical Services (PMS) practices or NHS authorities in the UK with the new contract for GPs.[15] Out-of-hours services ceased to be the responsibility of local GPs and were put out to tender. This was followed by the introduction of competition in in-hours primary care, with contracts under the arrangements for Alternative Provider Medical Services (APMS). APMS contracts do not need to be covered by the same transparency and oversight by PCTs and national quality assurance arrangements as in GMS practice,[16] such as the QOF. In contrast, APMS are intended to be freed from extensive rules that protect the public interest and to be based on 'light touch and low bureaucracy', in a climate where APMS franchise holders enjoy 'high trust'.[15] Furthermore, the Freedom of Information Act does not automatically extend to private business, while APMS and other contracts may be covered by 'commercial confidentiality',[17] potentially shrouding data on quality and costs from public and academic scrutiny. APMS practices can be bought and sold on the market, unlike conventional general practices.

Meanwhile, BBC TV journalists from *Panorama*, the investigative programme, reported in July 2008[18] that management consultants from US health corporations such as Aetna,[19] Humana[20] and UnitedHealth[21] were 'quietly flown in' to provide 'commissioning support to PCTs'. The UK government, Department of Health and NHS told *Panorama* they did not know how many advisers were present, while a number of PCTs only released the information after the BBC appealed on the basis of the Freedom of Information Act.[22] *Panorama* observed that there was nothing to stop the US corporations, as commissioning advisers, to recommend themselves for service delivery contracts. Companies such as Aetna[23] and UnitedHealth – or their daughter organisations – have indeed received service delivery contracts.

Heins *et al.*[16] studied the nature and extent of private provision, including APMS in primary care, using the Freedom of Information Act.[22] They observe that it is often difficult to characterise the nature of the bidding primary care providers, as traditional GP groups, cooperatives and other formally non-profit organisations band together with for-profits. Social Enterprises cover a range of business models, from paying out high salaries to owners and managers, leaving less for improving care, to prioritising improvement in clinical services over seniors' pay. Social Enterprises include Community Interest Companies (CICs)[24] that offer protection against asset stripping and require profits to be ploughed back into local services. In Birmingham, however, a CIC teamed up with a daughter organisation of Aetna, the giant US for-profit healthcare organisation.[23]

With the introduction of the Health and Social Care Bill in 2012,[25] England's health reform took a new direction. The bill proposes that groups of GPs decide on what care the bulk of the NHS budget will be spent, although the providers will have to be selected in processes that are prescribed by competition law and overseen by competition watchdogs.

In January 2011, an RCGP survey[26] found that 61% of GPs disagreed with the direction of the reforms, with 24% agreeing. More than 70% disagreed that competition between multiple providers would improve care outcomes or increase accountability in the NHS. After modifications and in spite of strong public and professional opposition legislation was passed by parliament in 2012,[27] completed by further arrangements on competitive tendering in 2013.

The King's Fund and the National Council for Voluntary Organisations observed that the 'new system is anything but a level playing field'.[28] Reynolds and McKee warned that the commissioning process has an intrinsic bias in favour of for-profit bidders including corporate giants with huge reserves and dedicated teams of lawyers and other experts preparing expensive tendering documents. Charities may not have the money and be unable to borrow for such exercises, unless certified by a third party that the loan is repayable without prejudicing its charitable activities, while NHS trusts that lose contracts run out of money and may have to close.[29]

....

Case scenario: commercialisation of primary care in Camden, London

In Camden, North London, contracts for four general practices have been
awarded to for-profit companies. In 2008, three went to UnitedHealth
UK, a subsidiary of the US health insurance giant. UnitedHealth UK is
headed by Simon Stevens, former health policy adviser to Tony Blair.
Three years later, the company sold its shares to another private provider
and one surgery at Camden Road closed in early 2012, surprising patients.
While the Chief Executive of North Central London NHS Trust said that
there was 'nothing to suggest that private providers are worse in any
way for patients', local GPs and a pharmacist raised concerns about the
fast turnover of locums, poor continuity of care and the loss of a nearby
surgery for patients with mobility problems.[30]

In 2009, another practice went to Care UK, headed by Dr Mark Hunt, who
previously worked in the Strategy Unit of the Department of Health.
Camden PCT did not wait until the public consultation on its primary
and acute care strategy was closed in October 2009. A group of concerned
citizens, including a former councillor and the Camden Keep Our NHS
Public pressure group, started court proceedings, alleging insufficient
consultation, leading to the suspension of Care UK's contract.[31]

....

Health care: a market or a service?

What are the issues in the commercialisation of primary care? Protagonists argue that patients choose providers on the basis of informed
choices and drive up standards as they opt for the best.[32] When money
follows the patient, healthcare organisations that fail to attract sufficient
customers lose funding and may go out of business. In this concept, front-
line health professionals are seen as having their own 'producer interests'
that need to be kept in check by managers and board members in NHS
institutions who are increasingly drawn from private enterprise.[33]

However, in most urban areas, patients can and do already choose
between a number of GP practices. Critics observe that patient choice is
not helped by government efforts to concentrate GPs in larger centres,
while in England it is commissioning organisations informed by English
and European Competition Law that choose which provider will be where
and for how long, and not patients or communities.

US economist Kenneth Arrow[34] put forward in 1963 that the delivery
of good health care is a service and incompatible with market principles.
Health care is characterised by asymmetry between doctor and patient in
terms of information and power, and by the inherent uncertainty regarding diagnoses and treatment. Also, contracts for care by insurers are

incomplete, as they cannot cover all eventualities. Arrow concluded that care must be based on trust: trust that the doctor has the best interests of the patient at heart. Subjecting it to markets and profits will lead to abuse of trust and the exploitation of patients. Arguably, uncertainty can be reduced but not removed by improving quality through clinical governance and accountability. Indeed, health professionals can improve their trustworthiness by adopting rigorous, enforceable medical ethics, and opening themselves up to scrutiny by patients, the public and experts.

For-profit commercialisation

Academics comparing the UK NHS with the heavily commercialised US[35] noted that primary care in the US is increasing overheads and draining resources. Academics, studying the social determinants of health for the World Health Organization, observed that there is no evidence that commercialisation offers benefits, in terms of cost or quality, over non-profit provision.[36] Devereaux et al.[37] studied costs in investor-led and non-profit hospitals in the US in a systematic review and meta-analysis. They concluded that for-profits were at least 19% more expensive. In the UK in 2007, private hospital providers received a premium of 11% over the NHS price, plus an undisclosed subsidy for bidding and other cost.[38]

Needleman[39] observed that, in the US, patient trust was reduced in for-profit healthcare organisations, providers and insurers, but that patients often did not know whether they were registered with a for-profit or a non-profit. For-profits are less likely to undertake community-oriented projects, such as treating destitute patients for free, or providing teaching and training. Those that do offer such services are often converted non-profits. For-profits engage more in untrustworthy activities such as 'upcoding' – phrasing claims in such a way that a higher fee can be obtained than is justified. Needleman also observed that non-profits behave very much like for-profits in highly competitive environments. Meanwhile, trust in individual health professionals remains remarkably robust in the US, especially when patients can choose their doctor. Mechanic, a health policy academic, summarised that patients want to see a doctor they know and trust,[40] and observed that good communication skills – attributes that are central to trust – can be learned.

Exploitation of patients

Risk profiles of individual patients and populations can be developed and linked to healthcare costs incurred by the same individuals or groups, forming the basis for not only the rational, equitable allocation of resources, but also the exploitation of patients for monetary gain. Different implicit or explicit processes can be applied by organisations and individual health professionals, including 'skimming, dumping and skimping'.[41,42] It involves taking on low-risk, low-cost patients and raising barriers for the registration of those who are likely to be costly; encouraging patients who require more resources to go somewhere else; and providing cheaper, sub-optimal care. Vulnerable patients are more likely to suffer as a result, including those with less education, those who are less articulate due to language barriers or other communication difficulties, those who are less assertive, and those without advocates. This can also happen in non-commercial settings and in conventional, partner-led primary care, when individual health professionals or organisations seek to reduce their workload. However, the introduction of large investor-led and other for-profit organisations may bring in new dimensions to organised exploitation.

Mechanic,[43,44] studying US Health Maintenance Organisations, predicted that cost control would 'depend more substantially on transfer of risk to providers, which keeps medical allocation implicit and more difficult to identify'. Mechanic sees this as a response to explicit denial of care in the US, which tends to infuriate the public. This development is – at least in part – reflected in incentive schemes for GPs in the UK aimed at reducing costs incurred by their patients through admissions and outpatient referrals. With a view to safeguarding equity and protecting vulnerable patients, continuous monitoring and data analysis will be required to help establish if skewing of results arises by referring patients to privately funded care and whether more assertive, articulate and higher-educated patients acquire better access to the detriment of more needy patients in the lower socioeconomic strata.

Tritter and colleagues[45] studied the UK, Finland and Sweden, and observed that the creation of healthcare markets is not driven by patients, for whom choice of provider – a keystone for the justification of markets – rarely tops their wish list. Business and ideology are more powerful forces, including the influence of multinational management consultancies that transfer ideas and approaches, and may also act as a broker between government and for-profit healthcare companies, according to emails made public following a freedom of information request.[46]

Drivers of health care

Two other areas may drive health care in England. First, government and its agencies, including NHS hospitals and PCTs, are subject to democratic control and the Freedom of Information Act.[22] Private companies are not, unless they are wholly owned by the government, while part of their activities may be covered by commercial confidentiality. Added to this are the effects of libel and defamation law, which are heavily skewed against individuals and small organisations with limited means. It doesn't only affect science and science journalism,[47] but also means that concerned citizens and small media organisations that seek to expose substandard care can relatively easily be 'gagged' by well-resourced organisations through injunctions and by the prospect of crippling legal costs for defendants.[48,49] Furthermore, organisations found to deliver poor care may not be deterred by the threat of large payouts to patients, as the UK does not have a US-style system of 'class actions', where groups of patients can much more easily obtain compensation through court action once fault has been established.[50]

Second, commercial interests may influence health care. This is acknowledged in rules regarding conflicts of interest in the English NHS, where more than a third of GPs on Clinical Commissioning Group (CCG) boards were found to have directorships or shares in private companies whose services CCGs could potentially commission.[51] More generally, there is the low threshold for politicians, political advisers, civil servants, but also doctors[52] to accept lucrative positions with companies whose paths they helped pave by their policies or action. In spite of the formulation of the Nolan principles on Standards in Public Life,[53] former secretaries for health, junior ministers, senior civil servants and government advisers have obtained multiple posts with corporations that operate within the orbit of the NHS, including Alliance Boots, CINVEN (a private equity company investing in private finance initiatives, including NHS infrastructure), BT that invests in NHS IT and many others.[54-58] MPs can similarly receive material support.[59] This situation, which is not unique to the UK, has its critics.[60] The US economist Robert Reich concludes that politics can be bought.[61] He sees this as a major barrier for equitable and sustainable economic, social and healthcare development. Reich proposes to separate politics from business and to promote the responsible citizen in us – a citizen who cares about his or her environment and the future, rather than a consumer chasing short-term gain. He proposes that former legislators and public officials be barred for at least five years from lobbying and a ban for business to fund political parties.

Doctors in leading or advisory positions can similarly be offered posts or establish their own companies. Huge financial interests may be at stake, as health care covers approximately one-tenth of our gross national product (GNP), our government intends to increase outsourcing[62] and, in time, up to 70% of the English healthcare budget may be managed by private companies.[38]

....

Question: what rules need to be established to guide politicians, civil servants and doctors, including staff of the NHS and the Department of Health, when they wish to take up lucrative posts in companies whose paths they helped pave?

....

Practice size, personal continuity and familiarity

Most primary care in the UK is delivered in practices served by a number of doctors, nurses, auxiliary and administrative staff, covering between 4000 and 7000 patients. In contrast, single-handed or two-doctor practices are still common in countries such as the Netherlands, France, Belgium and the US. Single-handed practices are highly rated by patients in both the UK[63,64] and the Netherlands,[65] and achieve similar scores in the UK on the clinical QOF indicators, if not better.[66] Smaller practices facilitate the development of familiarity[66] and personal continuity of care,[67-70] aspects highly appreciated by patients.[71] In contrast, the concentration of large numbers of doctors and patients can lead to the industrialisation[72] and commodification[73] of care, by reducing it to the sum total of discrete items that can be expressed in monetary terms, including consultation times, QOF scores, referrals and payments. Herein, health professionals may become interchangeable from one moment to another, and moved around and replaced with cheaper workers, as part of a 'flexible' labour force.

Consumerism and vulnerability in an unequal society

A key challenge is described by Martin Marshall in the 2009 RCGP James Mackenzie Lecture.[74] Marshall indicated that there are politically powerful critics of UK general practice, including a lead writer in *The Times* who thinks that the idea of a 'holistic approach' is a cloak for lack of expertise. The writer sees GPs as unnecessary as he uses them only to obtain referrals to specialists and prescriptions that he has decided he needs. Marshall warns that the GP profession fails to market its work and values.

Marshall's example resonates in the work of sociologist Richard Sennett,[75] who observes that, nowadays, political elites in Western societies see themselves not only as the deserving result of meritocracy but also as the norm for everyone else. What is good for them is good for others. Sennett contrasts this with the needs and wishes of many of those others, who have not been as 'successful' and who feel looked down upon. What is required first and foremost, according to Sennett, is respectful, personal and trusting relationships. The challenge, perhaps, lies in persuading elites and more consumerist patients to share the health service with those who have more personal and complex needs. This may be easier in Scotland and Wales, countries with stronger egalitarian traditions.

Confidentiality

Technological advances in care, fragmentation of care and advancing IT technology all call for and facilitate the easy recording and sharing of information about patients.[76] There are further developments, such as the Summary Care Record, which can be shared throughout the NHS by authorised persons, while research and healthcare planning are based on anonymised patient data.

Research[77] shows that patients often have the unrealistic expectation that only the health professional in the consultation sees their record. Davies[76] suggests that the Hippocratic notion of patient confidentiality no longer exists, observing that most guidance is more on when and how to break it than to maintain it. He proposes a thorough professional and public debate to redefine what confidentiality is, and what it is for.

Professional responses

How can GPs, registrars, their organisations and other members of primary care teams respond to these challenges and protect the position of vulnerable patients and disadvantaged groups? An aware-ness of the emerging differences between England on the one hand and Scotland, Wales and Northern Ireland on the other is essential. Role plays in registrar training and GP continuing education may be of help, where the different positions and roles of patients, doctors, owners or man-agers of for-profits and non-profits are explored. Here, the temptation can be offered to deliver substandard care to more needy, hence more costly patients, for the purpose of monetary gain for the organisation or the doctor.

Second, there is an urgent need to develop ethical guidance for con-flicts of interests between personal gain, the interests of commercial groups, and the protection of patients and communities, with enforce-able, credible sanctions for non-compliance. Professional organisations must be protected from becoming an arena where business goals are pursued. This could be helped by the requirement to publicly declare all interests at all times, and limiting the representation by GPs who are not mainly healthcare or academic practitioners, but businessmen and -women. Third, GPs must insist on the development of well-resourced quality assurance systems and institutions, including an inspectorate that is both authoritative and truly independent from politics, perhaps with a statute similar to the Judiciary. The inspectorate must have power and expertise to inspect and publish, overriding commercial confidentiality, and be equipped to withstand the libel lawyers. The Care Quality Commission, once stable, may form the basis for such an institution.[78] Fourth, GPs and their organisations in England could try to ensure, through CCGs and otherwise, that the statutory duty written in the Health and Social Care Act to reduce health inequalities[79] is adhered to. Best guidance could be used, as for instance in the case of vulnerable migrant women.[80] Care for disadvantaged groups of patients requires continuous monitoring of inequalities in healthcare provision and quality, and if necessary redistribution of resources within general practice and the health service as a whole.

Conclusion

General practice in the UK faces unprecedented challenges. England is moving away from the other countries in a more profit-oriented direction. Healthcare organisations that are owned by GPs or that employ GPs will be more driven by commercial motives. GPs needs a heightened awareness of how this may happen and how this can disadvantage their patients, in particular the most vulnerable. They need to be advocates and agents for corrective action on ethical and professional grounds.

Further reading

- Leys C, Player S. *The Plot against the NHS*. Pontypool: Merlin Press, 2011.

- RCGP Position on Health and Social Care Bill, www.rcgp.org.uk/policy/rcgp-policy-areas/health-and-social-care-reform.aspx [accessed July 2013].

References

1. Walt G. *Health Policy: an introduction to process and power*. London: Zed Books, 1996.

2. Department of Health. *Quality and Outcomes Framework*. London: DH, 2004, http://webarchive.nationalarchives.gov.uk/+/www.dh.gov.uk/en/Healthcare/Primarycare/PMC/Quality/OutcomesFramework/index.htm [accessed July 2013].

3. Doran T, Fullwood C, Kontopantelis E, *et al*. Effect of financial incentives on inequalities in the delivery of primary clinical care in England: analysis of clinical activity indicators for the quality and outcomes framework. *Lancet* 2008; **372 (l9640)**: 728–36.

4. Dixon A, Khachatryan A, Wallace A, *et al*. *Impact of Quality and Outcomes Framework on Health Inequalities*. London: King's Fund, 2011.

5. Roland M. The quality and outcomes framework: too early for a final verdict. *British Journal of General Practice* 2007; **57 (540)**: 525–7.

6. Heath I, Rubinstein A, Stange C. Quality in primary health care: a multidimensional approach to complexity. *British Medical Journal* 2009; **338**: b1242

7. McDonald R, Roland DM. Pay for performance in primary care in England and California: comparison of unintended consequences. *Annals of Family Medicine* 2009; **7(2)**: 121–7.

8. Organisation of Economic Cooperation and Development. Remuneration of doctors. 2009. www.oecd-ilibrary.org/social-issues-migration-health/health-at-a-glance-2011_health_glance-2011-en   [accessed July 2013].

9. Lester H, Campbell SM, McDonald R. The present state and future direction of primary care: a qualitative study of GPs' views. *British Journal of General Practice* 2009; **59(569)**: 908–15.

10. Kramer G. The ethics of payment for performance. *RCGP News*, 6 April 2011, 6.

11. Getz L, Sigurdsson JA, Hetlevik I. Is opportunistic disease prevention in the consultation ethically justifiable? *British Medical Journal* 2003; **327(7413)**: 498–500.

12. Hannon KL, Lester HE, Campbell SM. Patients' views of pay for performance in primary care. *British Journal of General Practice* 2012; **62(598)**: e322–8.

13. Ramesh R. £140 could buy private firms data on NHS patients. *Guardian*, 17 May 2013, www.guardian.co.uk/technology/2013/may/17/private-firms-data-hospital-patients?INTCMP=SRCH   [accessed July 2013]

14. Day M. UK government accused of privatising the NHS. *British Medical Journal* 2006; **333(7588)**: 61.

15. Department of Health. *Investing in General Practice: the new General Medical Services contract*. London: DH, 2003.

16. Heins E, Pollock AM, Price D. The commercialisation of GP services: a survey of APMS contracts and new GP ownership. *British Journal of General Practice* 2009; **59(567)**: e339–43.

17. Pollock A, Richardson L. Commercial confidentiality: a cloak for policy failure. *British Journal of General Practice* 2009; **59(569)**: 893–4.

18. NHS for Sale. *Panorama*, London: BBC TV, 7 July 2008, http://news.bbc.co.uk/1/hi/programmes/panorama/7487267.stm   [accessed July 2013].

19. Aetna, www.aetna.com.

20. Humana, www.humana.com.

21. UnitedHealth, www.unitedhealthgroup.com and www.unitedhealthuk.com.

22. Information Commissioner's Office. Freedom of Information Act. www.ico.gov.uk/what_we_cover/freedom_of_information.aspx   [accessed July 2013].

23. Anon. Public–private partnership reveals innovative approaches to improving health outcomes. *Alternative Providers*, 8 September 2009, http://alternativeprimarycare.wordpress.com/2009/11/11/aetna-uk/   [accessed August 2013].

24. Community Interest Companies, www.cicregulator.gov.uk.

25. Department of Health. *Equity and Excellence: liberating the NHS*. London: HMSO, 2010, www.official-documents.gov.uk/document/cm78/7881/7881.pdf   [accessed July 2013].

26. RCGP survey highlights GP concerns over NHS Reforms. 2011. www.rcgp.org.uk/news/2011/february/rcgp-survey-highlights-gp-concerns-over-nhs-reforms.aspx   [accessed July 2013].

27. *Health and Social Care Act.* London: TSO, 2012, www.legislation.gov.uk/ukpga/2012/7/contents/enacted [accessed July 2013].

28. Curry N, Mundle C, Sheil F, *et al. The voluntary and community sector in health: implications of the proposed NHS reforms.* London: King's Fund, 2011, www.kingsfund.org.uk/publications/voluntary_sector.html [accessed July 2013].

29. Reynolds L, McKee M. 'Any qualified provider' in NHS reforms: but who will qualify? *Lancet* 2012; **379(9821)**: 1083–441.

30. Foot T. Trust seeks legal advice to stop private firms selling GP practices. *British Medical Journal* 2012; **344**: e3993.

31. Foot T. Campaigners' clinic victory. *Camden New Journal*, December 2009, www.camdennewjournal.com/news/2009/dec/campaigners%E2%80%99-clinic-victory [accessed August 2013].

32. LeGrand J. The Blair legacy? Choice and competition in public services. Transcript of Public Lecture, London School of Economics, 21 February 2006, www2.lse.ac.uk/PublicEvents/pdf/20060221-LeGrand.pdf [accessed July 2013].

33. Pollock AM. *NHS Plc: the privatisation of our health care.* London: Verso, 2004.

34. Arrow KJ. Uncertainty and the welfare economics of medical care. *American Economic Review* 1963; **53**: 941–73, www.who.int/bulletin/volumes/82/2/PHCBP.pdf [accessed July 2013].

35. Dodoo M, Roland M, Green L. UK Lessons for US primary care. *Annals of Family Medicine* 2005; **3(6)**: 561–2.

36. World Health Organization. *Closing the Gap in a Generation: health equity through action on the social determinants of health. Final Report of the Commission on Social Determinants of Health.* Geneva: WHO, 2008, www.searo.who.int/LinkFiles/SDH_SDH_FinalReport.pdf [accessed July 2013].

37. Devereaux PJ, Heels-Ansdell D, Lacchetti C, *et al.* Payments for care at private for-profit and private not-for-profit hospitals: a systematic review and meta-analysis. *Canadian Medical Association Journal* 2004; **170(12)**: 1817–24.

38. Pollock AM, Godden S. Independent sector treatment centres: evidence so far. *British Medical Journal* 2008; **336(7641)**: 421–4.

39. Needleman J. The role of nonprofits in health care. *Journal of Health Politics, Policy and Law* 2001; **26(5)**: 1113–30.

40. Mechanic D. In my chosen doctor I trust. *British Medical Journal* 2004; **329(7480)**: 1418–19.

41. Barros PP. Cream-skimming, incentives for efficiency and payment system. *Journal of Health Economics* 2003; **22(3)**: 419–43.

42. Edwards N. Using markets to reform health care. *British Medical Journal* 2005; **331(7530)**: 1464–6.

43. Mechanic D, Schlesinger M. The impact of managed care on patients' trust in medical care and their physicians. *Journal of the American Medical Association* 1996; **275(21)**: 1693–7.

44. Mechanic D. The functions and limitations of trust in the provision of medical care. *Journal of Health Politics, Policy and Law* 1998; **23(4)**: 661–85

45. Tritter JQ, Koivusalo M, Ollila E, *et al. Globalisation, Markets and Healthcare Policy: redrawing the patient as consumer.* London: Routledge, 2010.

46. Spinwatch, 2011, www.scribd.com/doc/63941525/DH-Dalton-McKinsey-Correspondence [accessed July 2013].

47. Hurley R. The chilling effect of English libel law. *British Medical Journal* 2009; **339**: b4429.

48. Marcovitch H. Libel law in the UK. *British Medical Journal* 2009; **339**: b2759.

49. Verkaik R. Defame academy: the libel specialists. *Independent*, 7 July 2008.

50. Pallast G. *The Best Democracy Money Can Buy*. London: Pluto, 2002.

51. Iacobucci G. More than third of GPs on CCG boards have conflicts of interest. *British Medical Journal* 2011; **342**: d2216.

52. Pollock A, Price D. Privatising primary care. *British Journal of General Practice* 2006; **56(529)**: 565–6.

53. Committee on Standards in Public Life, www.public-standards.org.uk.

54. Anon. Executive profile: Patricia Hewitt. *Bloomberg Business Week*, http://investing.businessweek. com/research/stocks/private/person.asp?personId=42375726&privcapId=19685&previousCap Id=19685&previousTitle=Cinven%20Limited [accessed July 2013].

55. Wright O. Parliament ban for Hoon over 'cash for access'. *Independent*, 10 December 2010, www.independent.co.uk/news/uk/politics/parliament-ban-for-hoon-over-cash-for-access-2155936.html [accessed July 2013].

56. Walker K. Shamed 'cash-for-lobbying' MP Patricia Hewitt 'set to join Eurotunnel'. *MailOnline*, 26 March 2010, www.dailymail.co.uk/news/article-1260711/Shamed-cash-lobbying-MP-Patricia-Hewitt-set-join-Eurotunnel.html#ixzz1J37M81Uz [accessed July 2013].

57. Timmins N. Man at heart of NHS reforms moves to bank. *Financial Times*, 20 November 2006.

58. BMJ Informatica Company Team. Dr Mark Hunt. http://informatica.bmj.com/company/team/ mark-hunt/#.UgzVzW2t1SA [accessed August 2013].

59. Watt H, Prince R. Andrew Lansley bankrolled by private healthcare provider. *Telegraph*, 14 January 2010, www.telegraph.co.uk/news/newstopics/mps-expenses/6989408/Andrew-Lansley-bankrolled-by-private-healthcare-provider.html [accessed July 2013].

60. Milne S. A culture of corruption has seeped far into government. *Guardian*, 1 July 2009, www.guardian.co.uk/commentisfree/2009/jul/01/corruption-business-government-transport-health?INTCMP=SRCH [accessed July 2013].

61. Reich R. *Supercapitalism: the transformation of business, democracy, and everyday life*. New York: Alfred A. Knopf, 2007.

62. Timmins N. Outsourcing covers third of services. *Financial Times*, 9 July 2008, www.ft.com/ cms/s/0/e4b000da-4dea-11dd-820e-000077b07658.html#axzz1yQOjdu3z [accessed July 2013].

63. Campbell SM, Hann M, Hacker J, *et al.* Identifying predictors of high quality care in English general practice: observational study. *British Medical Journal* 2001; **323(7316)**: 784–7.

64. Baker R. Characteristics of practices, general practitioners and patients related to levels of patients' satisfaction with consultations. *British Journal of General Practice* 1996; **46(411)**: 601–5.

65. van den Hombergh P, Engels Y, van den Hoogen H, *et al.* Saying 'goodbye' to single-handed practices: what do patients and staff lose or gain? *Family Practice* 2005; **22(1)**: 20–7.

66. Roland M. Assessing the options available to Lord Darzi. *British Medical Journal* 2008; **336(7645)**: 625–6.

67. Schers H, van den Hoogen H, Bor H, *et al.* Familiarity with a GP and patients' evaluations of care. A cross-sectional study. *Family Practice* 2005; **22 (1)**: 15–9.

68. Baker R, Boulton M, Windridge K, *et al.* Interpersonal continuity of care: a cross-sectional survey of primary care patients' preferences and their experiences. *British Journal of General Practice* 2007; **57 (537)**: 283–9.

69. Mainous III A G, Goodwin M A, Stange K C. Patient-physician shared experiences and value patients place on continuity of care. *Annals of Family Medicine* 2004; **2(5)**: 452–4.

70. Mainous III A G, Baker R, Love M, *et al.* Continuity of care and trust in one's physician: evidence from primary care in the United States and the United Kingdom. *Family Medicine* 2001; **33 (1)**: 22–7.

71. Healthcare Commission. *Primary Care Trust Survey of Patients 2005.* London: Healthcare Commission, 2005.

72. Rastegar D A. Health care becomes an industry. *Annals of Family Medicine* 2004; **2(1)**: 79–83.

73. Leys C. The National Health Service. In: *Market-Driven Politics: neoliberal democracy and the public interest.* London: Verso, 2001, pp. 165–210.

74. Marshall M. Practice, politics, and possibilities. *British Journal of General Practice* 2009; **59 (565)**: e273–82.

75. Sennett R. *Respect in a World of Inequality.* New York/London: W.W. Norton & Company, 2003.

76. Davies P. Confidentiality: a contested value. *British Journal of General Practice* 2009; **59 (567)**: 718–19.

77. Greenhalgh T, Wood G W, Bratan T, *et al.* Patients' attitudes to the summary care record and HealthSpace: qualitative study. *British Medical Journal* 2008; **336(7656)**: 1290–5.

78. Timmins N. England's healthcare regulators will start 2010 without chiefs. *British Medical Journal* 2009; **339**: b5390.

79. Department of Health. *Equality Objectives Action Plan 2012–16.* London: DH, 2012, www.dh.gov.uk/health/2012/04/equality-objectives-2012-16/ [accessed July 2013].

80. Feldman R. *Guidance for Commissioning Health Services for Vulnerable Migrant Women.* London: Women's Health and Equality Consortium, 2012, www.whec.org.uk/wordpress/wp-content/uploads/downloads/2012/05/GuidanceCommissioningHealthServVulnMigrantWomen2012.pdf [accessed July 2012].

Index

Page numbers in italic refer to figures or tables.